Born At Risk

B. D. Colen

Also by the author:
Karen Ann Quinlan: Dying in the Age of Eternal Life

Born At Risk

B. D. Colen

Photographs by Linda Wheeler

St. Martin's Press
New York

Library of Congress Cataloging in Publication Data

Colen, B D
    Born at risk.

    1. Infants (Premature) 2. Infants (Premature)
—United States. 3. Infants (Premature)—Hospital
care—United States. 4. Neonatal intensive care—
United States. I. Title.
RJ250.C6   618.92′011   80-21579
ISBN 0-312-09291-1

Design by Deborah Horowitz
10 9 8 7 6 5 4 3 2 1
First Edition

This book is dedicated to all the infants born at risk, with the hope that someday the system of care described here will be standard for all such babies; and to Sara, Alicia, and Benjamin.

Acknowledgments

This is a work of nonfiction. The names of all persons and institutions, other than Children's Hospital National Medical Center and The Johns Hopkins Hospital, have been changed to protect the privacy of the individuals involved. But all the events described and the conversations repeated here actually took place. Some of them, however, did not occur in the chronological order in which they are reported.

The writing of a book such as this would have been impossible without the cooperation of literally dozens of individuals. First among them is the man I have chosen to call Dr. James Hannan, chief of neonatology at Metropolitan Lying-In Hospital, Washington D.C. Jim Hannan willingly allowed me into his nursery and his life, hoping that I would portray his still-infant medical specialty in such a way that it would be less foreign and more understandable to parents who encounter it after or while reading this book. All he asked in return was that I place in

viii

proper perspective whatever human frailties or medical mistakes I might observe. For this I am eternally grateful and hope he is not disappointed.

As Jim Hannan is quick to point out, a neonatologist alone cannot begin to provide the kind of care required by tiny, sick, premature newborns. Without a staff of highly trained, skilled, and dedicated nurses, there is no Intensive Care Nursery. And without the gracious cooperation of those nurses at Metropolitan Lying-In, this book could not have been written.

I would especially like to thank the parents who agreed to talk to me at length at a time in their lives when they were under great stress. They opened up their hearts and minds in the hope that other parents in similar circumstances could gain from reading about such an experience.

Thanks, too, are due my agent, Dennis Holler, and my editor at St. Martin's Press, Barbara Anderson, for their unflagging enthusiasm and support for this project. I could never have completed the book without their help.

Dr. John Scanlon, associate professor of pediatrics, Georgetown University School of Medicine, and Dr. Frank M. Midgely, assistant professor of surgery, George Washington University School of Medicine, reviewed the manuscript for technical accuracy, and for that I am deeply appreciative.

And last, but certainly not least, a special thank you to Paul W. Valentine, Douglas B. Feaver, and Donald E. Baker for a decade of professional guidance, personal advice, and, most important, true friendship.

B. D. Colen
May 3, 1980
Washington, D.C.

Introduction

Those who believe
Place dolls in Isolettes
For two-pound babies
To play with.
And you know,
It's a funny thing,
The two-pound babies
With the dolls in the Isolettes
Grow better.
        The babies of those who believe.

Born at Risk is a story of those who believe. Not religious men and women, not exceptionally erudite men and women, not even exceptionally gifted physicians—but believers. In a day and age when we abort our unborn, drug our teenagers, and place our old in warehouses, these are the surviving believers. The physicians who make continuous house calls in a day and age when no one makes house calls.

They are not gods, these physicians. They swear and bleed and sweat like the rest of us. They make mistakes. They are not always right. Frequently they are wrong, but for even the one-pound babies they try—with time and technique and heart—and that is what makes them different.

One could never say that as a group these physicians made money in Perinatal Medicine or that they bettered their academic careers by devoting huge quantities of time to critically ill infants. On the contrary, the surgeons make more money and the researchers get more credit.

One look at the divorce rate of this group would make you shudder. The burnout and turnover are high. Christmas Eve in the neonatal intensive care unit is not conducive to building good intrafamily relationships. But it is no accident that the author of this story set the time in the yuletide season. Where else is it always Christmas?

The number of infants lost per thousand livebirths in 1875 was one hundred twenty-five. Now in 1980 it is close to eighteen per thousand livebirths. To make this reduction, to save these infants, took an enormous quantity of time, effort and money. Society of course contributed much. Sometimes willingly, sometimes not. But it has only been recently that the believers were able to teach society that babies have the right to be born well and even to die well, that we should do our best for those who cannot ask for help and probably will never even know the physicians who gave it to them. It can be said that these physicians revolutionized our culture with this belief.

As a witness to the activity of the neonatal intensive care unit, Mr. Colen is exceptionally honest. He never glamorizes or giggles. He presents an almost photographic picture of the daily activities. The vignettes he describes are true-to-life and reflect Mr. Colen's background in journalism. The discussions, the frustrations, the love of the "frog," they're all there.

But there is more to the neonatal intensive care unit than the baby pictures posted on the walls or the sound of the beep-beep which permeates the unit. And that more is believing. It is the intense belief that it is good to live regardless of the effort it requires. The neonatal intensive care unit is not free. It is not pretty. But it is beautiful.

Rita G. Harper, M.D.
Chief,
Division of Perinatal Medicine
North Shore University Hospital;
Associate Professor of Pediatrics
    and Obstetrics and Gynecology
Cornell University Medical College

Preface

The first time I saw my one-day-old baby, lying in her incubator in the Intensive Care Nursery, an incredible sadness overwhelmed me. Three-pound Sarah Elizabeth, born in the twenty-eighth week of my pregnancy, looked more like a baby kitten than a baby human, her tiny red body and bony limbs covered with fuzzy dark hair. She had an IV inserted in her leg and she was hooked up to heart and respiration monitors by a maze of wires attached to plastic circles glued to her chest and leg.

She was certainly not the bouncing baby girl I had planned to deliver two months later, and a far cry from the nine-pound baby boy I had given birth to four years earlier.

I found it difficult to identify with the tiny creature in the glass box; to acknowledge her as my child. I felt I had somehow failed her, causing her to be born into a world she wasn't ready for, a world of bright lights and loud noises, a world that forced her to breathe, where people handled her and inserted tubes down her throat and stuck needles into her—a world so different from the peaceful, warm, dark, wet place inside me which she was entitled to call home for at least two more months.

I had been so happy with her inside me; and now I was so sad to have had her taken from me too soon.

Sarah was so small and her lungs were so immature that breathing problems or infections could pose threats to her life.

While the other mothers on the maternity ward had their babies with them in their rooms to feed and play with and hold, I had no one. While the other mothers would be bringing their new babies home with them when they left the hospital, I would be leaving alone. If my baby survived the first critical days after birth, it would be several weeks, even months, before she gained enough weight to come home.

Much has been written about the importance of infant-maternal bonding—that crucial contact between mother and newborn during the first minutes and hours after birth. I wondered what would happen to Sarah, lying alone in her glass house, with no one to hold her and love her. And I wondered what would happen to me, how I would make it through those months, without her.

For two months, I visited Sarah every day, sometimes twice a day, as if she were a prisoner in her glass cell. Sometimes I was able to hold her, to change her diaper and feed her, or just to stroke her body through the opening of her Isolette. Although I knew she was receiving the best possible care, it seemed like she belonged to the hospital, not to me.

I led a strange existence during those months. I was no longer pregnant, yet I didn't have a baby I could proudly show the world. Although I was bringing her my breast milk for her eight feedings a day, I had the freedom to go out whenever I wanted to, and to sleep as much as I wanted, with no night feedings, which mothers of newborns don't usually enjoy. Yet every time I saw a mother with an infant, I yearned for my own.

At night, when our little family was together, reading my son his bedtime books, I couldn't help but think of Sarah, lying alone in her incubator, hooked up to her monitors, under the constant bright lights of the ICN. And I cried for her, and for me.

As I look back now, a year later, I realize that it was my mistake to regard Sarah's premature birth as some kind of terrible tragedy. In fact, it has become a most remarkable victory—a victory of a tiny human being to accomplish many great feats: to breathe, to fight for life, to battle against an unknown but massive infection, to receive nourishment, to grow, to survive—when the odds weren't terribly great in her favor. And a victory, only one of many, for the skilled doctors and nurses who save thousands of these fragile lives every year.

Remembering those months when the hospital was Sarah's home and my second home, two of the resident neonatologists stand out in my mind. One was a woman with the most beautiful sad eyes that reflected her depth of concern and caring for those helpless babies. I was told that this doctor would break down and cry when any of the babies got sick or "went bad" as they used to say in the ICN.

The other resident was a jovial young man with a cherubic face whom I had often seen observe a two-pounder and laugh. I understand now what was in that laugh—it was a laugh of wonder, of amazement, that so tiny a creature had that spark of life to survive. And I can only imagine how fulfilling it must be to have the skill to maintain that spark.

Born at Risk faithfully recounts the challenges to the doctors and nurses who employ their enormous skill to save patients whose lives are literally in their hands. All parents, indeed all people who care about children, will find themselves living that experience through this remarkable book, just as I relived my own experience.

The depth of details involved in the hour-by-hour account of life and death in an ICN educate the reader on the advances in the practice of neonatology at its best, while the superb characterizations of the doctors, nurses, and parents provide a moving human drama.

As my daughter reached her first birthday, our own drama seems far behind us. She is so happy, so good-natured, so calm, so healthy, that it is, in fact, easy to forget where she spent the first eight weeks of her life.

I hope that, if premature babies have memories, Sarah has forgotten the painful part of those weeks—to be born too soon, to be born at risk, and to be forced to survive on her own in a world she wasn't quite ready for.

But I hope that, somehow, she will not forget the other side of her birth experience: the gentle hands, the smiling faces, the friendly voices, the warmth and caring of all the nurses and doctors whose dedication and skill and love brought her home to me.

I know I never will.

Shelley Gollust

Born At Risk

B. D. Colen

Chapter One

Seven A.M. The sun wasn't up yet and wouldn't be for another twenty-nine minutes. But Dr. James Hannan was up and had been for an hour, jogging, showering, shaving, gulping a cup of black coffee before leaving the still house. Christmas vacation had started yesterday for the kids, so Christie had no reason to get up. After twelve years of marriage and thousands of these mornings, she'd finally learned to take Jim at his word when he said, "Don't bother to get up; all I'll have is coffee, and there's no reason for us both to suffer."

In another quarter-hour Hannan would be in the parking lot behind Metropolitan Lying-In Hospital, and he used the few remaining moments in the quiet isolation of the three-year-old Datsun 280-Z to think about the day ahead. The first problem was that this wasn't just any Friday; it was Christmas Eve. Despite his cry of "Whale turds!" (one of his favorite expletives) when he'd noticed the schedule, he had only himself to blame,

1

for without realizing what he was doing, he'd blithely done his best to honor everyone else's vacation requests and had once again placed himself on clinical for the two weeks starting the Monday before Christmas. So in addition to his administrative and teaching duties as the hospital's Chief of Neonatology, Jim Hannan was also the senior man in the Intensive Care Nursery and the senior man on call at night for the two weeks. "How bad can it be?" he wondered as he drove. "It's already been one of the busiest weeks of the year. Three kids under 1,000 grams since Wednesday. St. Francis sitting on its ass about taking baby Fontain. Jesus! We've been waiting three days to get that kid over there to get her belly opened up and they keep farting around. The kid's mother's already lost three days of work sitting by the warming table waiting for the ambulance that doesn't come. Have to give Anna a call today and see if I can goose her into doing something. We've only got one unused respirator, and we're still full even after we transferred two kids back to the regular nursery. Well, at least I can be sure that what ever *can* go wrong, will."

Hannan's parking spot was empty, the 2 inches of fresh snow still unmarked, when the call came. It was 7:31. Mary Anne Nolan, nurse-coordinator on the day shift and the Code Pink nurse for the day, had barely gotten her coat off. "ICN. Nolan," she said, lifting the receiver.

"Ravi!"

Mary Anne heard laughter coming from the small, open, combination office-chart room between the two main rooms of the unit, but no response. "Javed! Oh- six!" Dr. Ravi Javed heard her and answered the phone.

"Javed here." He listened for about twenty seconds and then asked, "How many weeks is she? Twenty-nine? Have they done a sonogram? What complications? We're on our way." As a fully trained pediatrician doing two additional years' training in neonatology, Ravi Javed was in charge of the Code Pink team today. The team was always made up of at least a Fellow and two Intensive Care Nursery nurses and was supposed to be, but wasn't always, called to be on hand for all Lying-In's high-risk deliveries. And what was about to happen in Delivery Room 3 fit the criteria for a Code Pink.

As Javed dashed out the door of the nursery, Mary Anne grabbed the floral-patterned Code Pink bag from underneath the office counter and hurried along behind him, with Susie Phillips, the other RN on the team, running to catch up. Javed was at the stairwell door, about 100 feet from the fourth-floor unit, before the women caught up with him. "What have we got?" asked Mary Anne, as the three of them clattered down the ancient stairs, an infinitely faster route to the first floor than what were jokingly referred to as the elevators. "Probably a twenty-nine-weeker," Javed replied, panting slightly. "The mother's been in-house for a week; came in when her membranes ruptured at home. Martinez tried to hold her off, but he can't any longer."

"Why wasn't she on the board?" asked Mary Anne, realizing as she asked it that it was a silly question, given that only about a quarter of the hospital's obstetricians ever bothered to inform the ICN when they had a high-risk mother in the hospital. So the "In-house" blackboard in the unit was some help, but not enough. "When will they learn?" wondered the nurse. "A baby's got enough problems arriving two or three months early without arriving like some extra dinner guest when it isn't expected." It was something she'd thought about so often that thinking it was almost as much a part of a Code Pink for her as grabbing the flowered bag.

Javed, the first of the three out of the stairwell, hit the red button on the wall and the double wooden doors to the delivery area swung open, almost clipping Susie, who was thinking about Christmas and not the fact that the doors swing out. The three shed the gowns they had pulled over their surgical scrubs, tossing them in the laundry hamper just inside the doors to the delivery suite. They pulled on their booties, caps, and masks, with Javed pulling on a full head arrangement that covered his beard as well as his hair. Before adding his mask he looked like a knight in disposable paper chain mail.

Ninety seconds after receiving the Code Pink call, the team was in Delivery Room 3, where final preparations were underway for baby McKnight's delivery. Lucy McKnight, nineteen, single, unemployed, black, and scared, lay on the delivery table in the center of the green-tiled room, her feet already strapped into the stirrups, her dignity left behind in the labor room. Always an echo chamber, the delivery room was particularly noisy now, as Javed and his team set up and checked their equipment in the corner to the right of McKnight's feet. The head delivery room nurse checked the OB instruments, each with its own peculiar clatter and clang, while Dr. Emilio Martinez readied himself for the delivery.

"I need a chair," Martinez announced to no one in particular. But Betty Rogers, who had been with the chief of Lying-In's medical staff through more deliveries than she cared to count, had the black vinyl seat of an OR stool beneath the pale green seat of Martinez's scrubs before the verbalized thought could become a command. "This isn't the one I'm used to," he said. "Do we have one with a back on it?"

"No, doctor," replied Betty, just as she always answered the stock question.

"Oh, well." He settled himself on the stool. "Have we got some Xylocaine?" He was handed a hypodermic of the local anesthetic. "Mrs. McKnight?" He was seated between the woman's legs, but with the clatter in the room and her contractions, he wasn't at all sure of being heard. "Can you hear all right, Mrs. McKnight?"

Lucy McKnight mumbled "Yes" between moans.

"We're just going to give you a little oxygen, for the baby," he told the woman, who was trying to ask why a transparent green plastic mask was being fitted over her mouth and nose. "We're not going to put you to sleep." McKnight gasped sharply. "Are you having a contraction?" She nodded. "All right, I'm going to give you something here to deaden your nerves," said Martinez, readying the Xylocaine. "You'll feel a little stick. You can push if you like." Then, to the nurse standing by McKnight's head he said, "She can push," as though McKnight herself weren't there. "Can you push?" the nurse asked. "Take a deep breath, hold it, and push again."

"You can push," Martinez told McKnight. "You have a few pushes to make." He commented over his shoulder to Javed, "It's hard for her to tell what's what. It's her first baby. She can push it out in the bed or she can sit here and it'll take a while. At least she hasn't had any medication, other than the Xylocaine to deaden the nerves in the vaginal area."

"Now, Mrs. McKnight, do you hear me? Let's see you push down and have a feeling for it."

"Push down hard," coached the nurse.

"Do you have a contraction now?" asked Martinez. "No? Well, if you have one now I think we can do it in one or two pushes."

"Are you having one now?" asked the nurse. McKnight grimaced and nodded slightly. "Push down!"

"That's right," Martinez encouraged her. "That's it. Push down." The top of the baby's head was visible. "You can make it on the next push." McKnight, who had had no preparation for childbirth and didn't know anything about controlling her breathing to stay on top of the pain of the contractions, was yipping like an injured puppy. Her cries were the only sound for about thirty seconds.

"You can make it now if you just push once more. Easy, easy, push gently. Easy does it! You don't want it to come too fast. Easy, easy. It's coming. Just a minute! No good." Martinez's tone changed completely. It was now hard, one of command, not gentle coaxing. The baby's head had emerged, but so had two turns of the umbilical cord, wrapped tightly around the tiny neck. Martinez quickly clamped off the cord at both points where it emerged from the vagina and cut off the portion around the infant's throat. He then grabbed the baby and pulled it out. "I think it's a girl, at least it is in the last book I read!" he called to Lucy McKnight, who smiled slightly through the pain.

Mary Anne Nolan plucked the baby from Martinez's hands so quickly it seemed he had never held it, and almost as quickly the room was dominated by the sounds of the tiny infant being resuscitated. Karen Fitzgerald, the resident on the Code Pink team, had come in late, but she was there before the baby was born and it was she who was intubating the infant, forcing a tube down its trachea for connection to a hand respirator. Javed took the respirator, a black rubber bag the size and shape of a football with a flow valve attached, and hooked it to the inserted tube. He began pumping vigorously, the respirator making a noise similar to that of a hand bicycle pump. Lucy McKnight, hearing the noise but no baby's cry, strained to see her child. "It's a girl," Martinez told her again. "It's about two and a half pounds. It's small," he added, redundantly. With the tube for breathing properly inserted, a baby cannot cry. But no one had taken the time to explain that to Lucy McKnight.

"What's the heart rate?" asked Javed.

"I can't tell with you bagging," replied Susie, for whom this was her first Code Pink.

"They're resuscitating the baby," Martinez told the worried mother. He did not even look up from between her legs, where he was assisting her in delivering the placenta.

Betty Rogers stepped over to the stainless-steel intercom on the wall and hit the Delivery Suite nursing station button: "Hello? Could someone bring back one-sixth of MS, please?" Mary Anne, standing beside the warming table—a flat, waist-high unit with a heating element suspended above it, making it possible to work on the baby and maintain its body temperature without keeping it covered—began to suction the baby, clearing a yellowish secretion from its lungs. The noise, not unlike that of a vacuum cleaner in a puddle, startled Lucy McKnight.

"Just relax," Martinez told her. "Sometimes something gets caught in there." The noise of the suction was followed by a gurgling noise from the baby, and then, three minutes and twenty seconds after her birth, little girl McKnight tried to cry for the first time. The baby lay on her back on the table, looking exactly like a fetus in one of those photographs the Right-to-Lifers always display. Mary Anne turned to Susie and told her, "We'll need the Cavitron, and I think we're going to need the elevator in a little bit."

"Did you turn on the warmer and the battery?" she asked Susie when the trainee returned. "Not the red switch, the warmer and the battery? Okay."

"He doesn't look real pale now," Javed told the team. He continually referred to the female baby as "he." "He did look real pale, but he doesn't now."

"Can I have a clamp for the cord?" Mary Anne interrupted, telling Javed, "We may need a catheter."

"He looks real pink," Javed said, repeating himself.

"Do you want to reduce to 40 percent oxygen?" Mary Anne asked. "What do we want this baby on, a heated table?"

"Oh yeah, a heater," Javed agreed.

"And a respirator standby. What type, Bourns? Susie, push number seven," Mary Anne ordered, and Susie pushed button seven, the direct line to the ICN. "Hello?" called Mary Anne, not waiting for a reply. "We're going to need a heating table and a volume Bourns."

"A volume Bourns?" asked the hollow voice from four floors above.

"Right!"

Susie was trying to figure out what to do with the baby's iden-
tification bracelet, which was ludicrously large for the infant on
the table. "With some of these babies we just send the bracelet
upstairs," Mary Anne told her.

"I don't want it to get lost," Susie explained.

Mary Anne turned to Javed. "I'm going to get the Cavitron set
up. What IMV do you want?"

"IMV of thirty, pressure of twenty, fifty percent oxygen and
PEEP of five." As he finished ordering the settings for the oxygen
and monitoring parameters on the machine that would be used
to transport the baby, one of the Delivery Room nurses told
Javed, "When you get done, the mother would like to know
something about the baby."

"Mrs. McKnight? It's a baby girl," Javed began. "She wasn't
breathing initially—she was blue—so we had to breathe for her
by tube, and now she is looking pink and she's breathing on her
own all right. But we still have a tube in her to help her, okay?"
McKnight clearly didn't know whether it was or was not all
right. "I don't know her exact weight, but she looks like three
pounds. We'll tell you later what it is."

"Can I see her?" the mother asked plaintively.

"You can't see her right now, but when we've finished with
her, you'll be able to see her, okay? Otherwise, she seems to be in
pretty decent shape right now. She's small and it's hard to tell
what will happen in the next couple of days, but she is in pretty
decent shape now."

"She wasn't breathing?" asked Lucy McKnight. It was her first
question about the condition of her baby, whose birth was more
than ten weeks early.

"That's right," Javed told her.

Martinez expanded the succinct reply, explaining, "All babies,
when they're born, even the full-size ones, are a little bit blue.
Then they get pinker as they start breathing. But she's a premature baby, you know—she's ten weeks early—and this is as much

a surprise to her as it is to you. They're not always in the best shape to start functioning outside the uterus."

"How's the heart?" McKnight asked.

"The heart's all right," Martinez said. He continued: "The main thing is the breathing, the lungs. It's always the lungs, or almost always."

"She came out in pretty decent shape," Javed said. "She had the cord around her neck twice, but she looks pretty pink right now."

"She does look good now," Martinez reassured his patient. "I'd say two and a half pounds. If everything goes well, it's going to be about five or six weeks before she goes home. But that's just guessing off the top of my head right now. But she'll get the best of care. The neonatologists have the ball now."

The conversation was interrupted by Mary Anne, who had just wheeled in the Cavitron infant transporter. The unit contains a respirator; air compressor and blender; oxygen supply; its own electrical supply; lights; monitors for heart, respiration, and central venous pressure; and a heating element over the top in a curved, clear plastic cover, similar to the defroster unit in the windshield of a 747 jet. The baby can be observed through the radiant heating element, and the curved cover can be slid out of the way enough for the team to reach under the edge to work on the baby and, at the same time, keep the baby warm.

"We have a one-to-two IE ratio, Peak of twenty, PEEP of five, getting about fifty percent oxygen right now, okay?"

"All right, let's get her moved," said Javed, who watched as Karen Fitzgerald lifted the baby off the table and placed her into the Life Island. Seventeen minutes after she was born not breathing, baby girl McKnight was ready to leave for the nursery.

"All right, let's go," said Javed. "Is the oxygen set?"

"You have five hundred pounds," Mary Anne replied. "You can take your time."

"Thank you, everybody," Javed told the delivery room staff,

and the baby was wheeled over to the side of the table on which Lucy McKnight still lay. "Here's the baby," Javed told the mother. "We're helping her to breathe, see? Her eyes are open."

There were tears streaming down McKnight's cheeks as she saw her baby for the first time, a baby she thought she was going to lose. A nurse propped her up for a better look and she reached a hand out toward the Cavitron. "Little girl," was all she softly said to the baby who could not hear her.

"It's not quite equal to your uterus," Martinez said of the Life Island, "but it's the next best thing."

As the Code Pink team wheeled the Cavitron toward the waiting elevator, Javed remarked, "It's a Cadillac. It's too good for Lying-In."

"You mean it's too good for us?" Susie asked earnestly.

"It's too," he teased.

"Listen," said Fitzgerald, who had just finished a rotation at Suburban General (like Lying-In, one of St. Francis' teaching hospitals), "the only transport we have at General is our arms."

The elevator doors opened at the fourth floor and the Cavitron was rolled down the hall with Javed pulling and the women pushing and guiding it. Past the nursing station on the right. Past Jim Hannan's office on the left. Past the sign reading "Premature Nursery: Authorized Personnel Only," a holdover from the days when parents weren't welcome in the nursery twenty-four hours a day, as they are now. Up to the door marked 445, which Javed swung open with a trumpet-like "Ta-Da!" announcing the arrival of baby girl McKnight to the day shift. Two of the nurses rushed up to the new arrival. "Oh, she's got the nicest eyes!" gushed Kim Lee, at whom the baby seemed to be staring. "And she's got such a long cord."

The Cavitron was wheeled into the far corner of the room to an empty warmer, which had already been turned on. A blue Bourns Life Support Infant Respirator stood by the warming table, as did thirty-four pieces of equipment and surgery kits, everything in readiness from stethoscopes, to preweighed diapers, to a spare oxygen valve for the respirator, to 2×2 bandages. "What's the one-minute Apgar?" asked Arlene Hollins, the head nurse on the day shift, who with what seemed a single motion lifted the baby from the transporter onto a scale—2 pounds, 13 ounces—and back into the Cavitron.

"Give her a one for heart rate," replied Mary Anne. "Somebody give me some parameters. What do you want her on? Forty percent oxygen?"

"Hurry up and get her on the ventilator before she gets better," joked Hannan, who had arrived at the hospital a few minutes after the Code Pink call. Javed had taken the infant out of the Life Island and laid her on her back on the warming table.

"Wait a minute!" commanded Mary Anne, turning on the Fellow. "If we don't have the respirator set up, don't grab the baby from the transporter." Karen Fitzgerald bagged the baby with the hand respirator while Javed adjusted the Bourns. "God," thought Mary Anne, "it's enough of a chore having to teach the new nurses without having to go through this with the new Fellows all the time. They're supposed to know better, but after six months in here, any of my girls knows more than they do about how to handle an admission." There was some truth to what she was thinking, for in many hospital specialty units, adult as well as pediatric, the nursing staff does the fine tuning, watching the patients for the subtle changes missed by the new physicians, and teaching the daily routine of the unit.

"Do we have a girl McKnight?" asked Arlene Hollins, comparing the baby's bracelet with the chart.

Susie bent over and looked at the tiny infant. "Yup! It's baby McKnight and she is a girl."

"First things first," said Javed. "Let's get a Logan bar." The Logan bar is the frame used to steady the respirator tube when it is kept in the baby's throat for any but brief periods. The sides of the baby's head were swabbed with Benzoine to make the skin sticky and mole skin was used to hold the frame in place. The tube protruding from the infant's throat was no bigger than a standard drinking straw; an adult tube is as big as a small garden hose. The job of hooking up the respirator was completed, and Fitzgerald turned her attention to attaching the baby's monitor leads. She got the three leads to stick to the infant's chest on the first try but then made the mistake of trying to reposition one. After four tries she gave up and Javed took over. Susie then took the baby's temperature by placing an electronic thermometer under the infant's scrawny arm. It was 96.9 degrees. The warmer was turned up.

"Are you and Mary Anne going to admit this baby?" Hollins asked Susie.

"I think so," said the new nurse.

"Mary Anne, are you going to admit this baby?"

"Yes."

"All right then, what time does your primary-care baby get fed?"

"Eight-thirty."

"All right," said Hollins. "I'll take care of it."

Baby McKnight began fussing. Not crying, fussing. One of the first things that strikes visitors to the ICN is how little crying there is. Two reasons are the incredible amount of time the babies spend sleeping and the fact that most are in incubators. A third reason is that a baby whose endotracheal tube has been inserted properly cannot cry. "Hold on, you poor little thing," Mary Anne said softly to the fidgeting baby. "It's okay." She adjusted the temperature of the warming table upward.

"Don't overshoot the temperature," Javed warned. "The skin temperature's higher than it was, so if the baby's warming, don't adjust it yet."

"Do you want to start an IV?" Mary Anne asked, changing the subject.

"I want to put in a catheter first. And we need gastric culture, ear cultures, umbilical culture, everything."

"You don't need to order the cultures. We do them standard."

"I'm not talking standard; I'm talking about what I want to do in addition to standard," Javed told her.

"Oh my God," thought Mary Anne. "This is not what I need on Christmas Eve." But she also knew better than to respond to Javed's dig, and instead she explained to Susie that the cultures were being ordered to see whether the infant had picked up any infections during the week between the rupturing of its mother's membranes and its delivery.

Susie was struggling with a sound amplification system for listening to the baby's pulse. She was getting nothing but scratchy noise. "Let me do it, Susie," said Mary Anne, taking over. Within moments the corner of the room was filled with a rhythmic sound exactly like that of a submarine's sonar: the amplified sound of the blood rushing through baby girl McKnight's veins.

"Do we have blood here?" Javed asked.

"It's right here," said Karen Fitzgerald. She held up a bag containing 50 ccs of blood.

"Should we do the catheter and get it in?" asked Mary Anne.

"Right," said Javed. "Twenty is low blood pressure. It should be about twenty-five in a baby this size."

"Are you planning to get a catheter in?" asked Hannan, who had come back to check on things again and seemed annoyed that they were going so slowly. Javed was not one of his favorites. The senior man did not consider his junior particularly sharp or resourceful, and he had little use for people who were not both, a feeling he hid with great difficulty.

"Right," Javed told him. "We're going to give the blood and get the catheter in."

"Okay. I'll be in my office. If you guys need anything you can page me," said Hannan, who then left the nursery.

The team began preparing the baby for her transfusion, first taping a board to her left arm for the IV insertion. The 3½-inch board reached from the baby's hand to her elbow. "Can you hold this thing for me?" Javed asked everyone and no one. "I'll get the IV in." He took the hollow needle, the size of a small sewing needle, and probed for a vein in the infant's extended arm. After six tries he finally found a vein. "Let me have the tape for the butterfly, please," he told Susie, who looked at him as though he were speaking in his native dialect.

"Just yell out when you need things," said Mary Anne, whose patience was being sorely tried. "Susie doesn't know where things are yet, so just yell."

"Has the blood been checked?" the Fellow asked.

"It's checked. You can go ahead," she told him. Javed began pushing in the blood, initially giving the infant 15 ccs to get her blood volume, and therefore her pressure, up.

"Do me a favor," he said to Mary Anne. "Cut off the rest of the umbilical, clean it up, and recheck the temperature, and then we'll have to restrain the baby."

Mary Anne took care of the first two tasks and then she and Fitzgerald restrained the 15-inch baby by tying her hands and feet to the sides of the warming table with gauze strips. "She's too pink. If I put the catheter in now, it'll be a disaster," said Javed. "I have the shakes."

"Are you still hung over from that St. Francis party?" asked Nolan. Javed did not reply.

The baby's stomach and chest were swabbed with Betadine, an antiseptic to prevent infection, and she was then completely draped in pale green surgical towels, with only the stump of her umbilical cord exposed. "Is the baby restrained all fours?" Javed asked instead of looking

"Yes," Mary Anne replied flatly.

"I want to clean up this umbilical stump before I do the job," Javed explained, "so I don't have to worry about contamination there. Most people do it afterwards, but I'd rather do it first."

"We always do it first," Mary Anne told the Fellow, who had just come over to Lying-In from St. Francis three weeks earlier.

Javed's insertion of the umbilical catheter was far smoother than his fumbling with the IV, and in one swift move, he had the minute catheter inserted in the even smaller umbilical artery, allowing the nurses to draw arterial blood for blood gas workups with a simple twist of a stop cock and insertion of a hypodermic.

It was 8:37, one hour and six minutes after the Code Pink team had been called. Baby girl McKnight, 2 pounds 13 ounces of baby born ten weeks early, was established in the Intensive Care Nursery of Metropolitan Lying-In Hospital. If she survived the next twenty-three hours without serious complications, the odds were overwhelming that she would survive. Had she been born almost anywhere else in the city, it is likely she would have gone directly from the Delivery Room to the morgue. For had there been no Code Pink team at the delivery, she would never have begun breathing.

Chapter Two

"Any messages for me?" asked Jim Hannan, as he walked into his office.

"Just that Mr. Daniels, from *The Washington Post*. He asked me to have you call him back as soon as you got in," said Rita Andrews, Hannan's secretary.

"He'll have to wait. I don't want any calls or anybody coming in for the next five minutes." He hung out his red plastic "Do Not Disturb" sign, covering the hand-lettered notice, "Ogre at Work. Disturb at Your Own Risk!" that always hung on the wooden door. Even with the door closed, Hannan's office was not much larger than a good-sized storage closet. There were none of the trappings of rank formally associated with hospital or medical school department chairs: no mahogany desk with leather desk pad, no coffee tables or reproductions of DaVinci anatomical drawings, no sets of antique medical instruments, and no comfortably worn Oriental rug, but worn yellow carpeting covering the linoleum floor. At best, functionalism prevailed: a tired-looking yellow leatherette couch; a blue steel filing cabinet—the exposed side of which was plastered with notices of fishing and bird hunting awards Hannan had won and photos of Hannan proudly displaying trout and bass that didn't get away—and a book case crammed with textbooks on neonatology, pediatrics, obstetrics, pharmacology, mathematics, experimental design, and anatomy. "If You Take It out, Sign It Out!" ordered a note taped to the book case in an almost hopeless attempt to keep the expensive texts from walking away.

The desk at which Hannan sat was no fancier—institutional brown metal, not even matching the filing cabinet. Like all the other movable objects in the room, it bore a small metal plate engraved with a number and the words "Property of Metropolitan Lying-In Hospital." The right side of the desk was shoved against a wall covered with the framed tangible evidence of Hannan's fourteen years as a physician: the Boston University Medical School diploma, dated 1965; the certificates attesting to the completion of three successful years of general pediatric residency at the Massachusetts General Hospital, the two years in the U. S. Public Health Service—the "yellow berets," service in a community health clinic in a Spanish-speaking neighborhood of south Boston, the three years as a Fellow in neonatology at Boston Lying-In Hospital and Boston Children's, and the year as chief of Newborn Intensive Care at Boston's Beth Israel Hospital; and the certificates of appreciation for week-long stints in visiting professorships at various medical schools around the country. And all of it, he would think from time to time, "didn't mean shit" if it didn't help you save a particular baby at a particular time.

As he worked at his desk, Hannan could look up and see the blackboard at the far end of the room. Most of the scribbles and notations on the large board could be erased on a whim or the need for more space, but one column of notes running down the left-hand side of the board was guarded with the notation "Do

Not Erase." For here was the list of projects, papers, book chapters, and books that Hannan and members of his staff were currently working on: a behavioral study that Christie Hannan, Jim's wife and a nurse, was conducting for an internationally known pediatric behaviorist; a chapter Mary Anne was writing for a new nursing text; a drug study being conducted in the nursery; several book chapters Jim Hannan was working on; a paper due for submission by Tom Watkins to a professional journal; and so on. The parent of a baby in the nursery could read the list at any time and honestly think, "Other children will benefit from my baby's being here." Small consolation, no doubt, but consolation none the less.

Working by the light that even on a snowy winter day flooded through the windows along the southern wall of the office, Hannan flipped open the silver metal cardex file that lay before him on the desk. Within the twin aluminum covers lay the distillation of his knowledge about the condition of each of the twenty babies in the nursery down the hall—seventeen of them on intensive care status and three in the step-down, "high risk" unit, from which they would be discharged home or back to one of the hospital's regular nurseries.

The twenty 3 × 5 cards, sheathed in clear plastic and arranged in two columns of ten overlapping cards each, told as much about the mission and state of the art of neonatology as they did about each of the tiny babies whose medical histories they outlined. Hannan would normally be reading and editing these mini-charts during morning rounds, which would begin in a few moments. But he had been out of town at a medical meeting for the past three days and wanted to refresh his memory before taking on the Fellows, resident, and students in the nursery. He began flipping through the cards, pausing first when he came to baby Fontain. "Jesus!" he thought. "Poor little Becky. What in hell are we going to do with you?" Becky was the nursery's little old lady, born ninety-three days earlier at 740 grams (1.6 pounds). Now she weighed only 1,720 grams (3.8

pounds) and didn't seem to be gaining any weight. She had been on and off the respirator more times than Hannan cared to count. She'd managed to overcome a staph infection and a bout of sepsis, a general, system-wide bacterial infection. She was treated with indomethacin, a drug Hannan had been using successfully to treat babies whose patent ductus failed to close. Prior to the development of indomethacin, surgery had been, and sometimes still was, required to shut the passage between the aorta and pulmonary arteries, serving in the fetus to circulate the blood while bypassing the nonfunctioning lungs. The ductus is supposed to shut down itself within a few days of birth, but sometimes, particularly in premature babies, or premies, it fails to do so—thus the need for indomethacin. Hannan thought he had arranged to have Becky transferred to St. Francis for a surgical workup and possible corrective surgery for what he suspected was some kind of blockage of her esophagus preventing her from getting enough nourishment. But three days later, Becky was still lying on a warming table in the nursery.

Andrew Greene had been in Hannan's cardex for thirty days. Born weighing 2,000 grams (4.4 pounds), he had gained 2 pounds. He had suffered from idiopathic respiratory syndrome, referred to as respiratory distress syndrome in the nursery and known to the general public as hyaline membrane disease, one of the most common diagnoses in an intensive care nursery. The condition, which can cause the infant to suffocate if breathing isn't mechanically aided, is caused by a lack of pulmonary surfactant, a biochemical material that affects the surface tension of the aveoli, the tiny grapelike sacs that make up the lung. If there isn't enough surfactant, the aveoli collapse too far when the baby exhales and fail to expand when he tries to take the next breath. Baby Greene was placed on a mechanical respirator, or ventilator, to treat his respiratory distress syndrome, but he then developed a condition called bronchopulmonary dysplasia, a disease that appears to be the result of treatment. Although its precise cause is a matter of debate in the medical community, BPD, as it is known to the nurses and physicians who treat it, is a stiffening of the lung tissue resulting in breathing difficulty in some infants who are on respirators for protracted periods of time. Dispute arises over whether the condition is caused by high concentrations of oxygen, which must be forced directly into the lungs to treat the respiratory distress syndrome, or by the mechanical battering on the lungs from the force of the respirator as it pumps air down the endotracheal tube into the lungs. In addition to all his other problems, baby Greene had septicemia, a general systemic infection, and an abcess on his right hand—the abcess caused by one of the many IV needles attached to his body.

Hannan passed over Robert Morrison's card with barely a glance. Born a week earlier weighing 1,400 grams (3 pounds), baby Morrison had slipped to 1,370 grams, which was to be expected in the first week. Other than his size, his only problem thus far was a mean-looking cut on his neck caused by a slip of the obstetrician's knife during the emergency cesarean delivery. But he was doing well, breathing room air on his own with no sign of respiratory distress.

Shaunta Odell was another baby who was doing surprisingly well. Born weighing 1,088 grams (2.4 pounds), she had lost only 30 grams in the first week and now appeared to be gaining weight. She had had some respiratory distress and had been put on a respirator. She was still on the respirator but was now breathing room air rather than air supplemented with extra oxygen. "You'll do all right," thought Hannan, "if we can just get you off the ventilator soon enough." He flipped to the next card, Susan Breslin.

Susie was one of the nurses' favorites. Despite being born weighing 1,390 grams (3 pounds) in her mother's thirty-fifth week of pregnancy, Susie had gained a full pound in her three weeks in the middle of the nursery's three rooms. She had suffered from respiratory distress syndrome, which is most common in infants born between the thirty-second and thirty-fourth week of gestation. But she had come off the respirator two days before Hannan left on his trip and appeared to be doing well. Her mother made the 50-mile round-trip drive to the hospital at least once, and sometimes twice a day, to hold, touch, and just watch her baby for a few cherished hours. Her father, too, visited nearly every day.

"We're gonna have to keep a close eye on you today, kid," Hannan thought as he turned to Kizzie Lincoln's card. Kizzie was eight days old and weighed 1,400 grams (3.1 pounds), 33 grams less than she had weighed at birth. She had had some respiratory distress, which seemed to be under control. But when he had stuck his head in the nursery earlier in the morning, Hannan had been told Kizzie was jittery, and he knew what that meant. Roberta Lincoln, Kizzie's nineteen-year-old mother, had a seizure disorder and had been taking prescribed phenobarbital throughout her pregnancy. Kizzie had been born with Apgars of 2 at one minute and 5 at five minutes—out of a possible 10 each time—and the nursery staff assumed that her heart rate and respiration were depressed by the drug her mother had been taking. The Apgar score is a system used to measure the newborn's respiratory and neurological function. The jitteriness, Hannan knew, indicated that Kizzie Lincoln was starting to go through phenobarbital withdrawal and would have to be observed especially closely throughout the next twenty-four hours.

Sam Fisher, whose card was the next Hannan scanned, was still in rocky shape. Baby Fisher had entered the nursery six weeks earlier, weighing 740 grams (1.6 pounds), the second-born of a set of twins. Twin "A" had died shortly after birth, but Sam, who, ironically, was the smaller twin, had done beautifully for the first two days, breathing without the aid of a respirator his second day. But by the morning of the third day he had developed respiratory distress syndrome, which quickly became severe. He was still on the respirator six weeks later, but now he had a strep infection and BPD to add to his difficulties. Hannan hoped the infant would turn the corner, but things were still touch and go.

As he glanced at baby Smith's card, Hannan slowly shook his head. Darleeta was one month old on this Christmas Eve, and her mother had not visited her once in the past thirty days. Medically, Darleeta had been "one sick little girl," Hannan thought. Born weighing 880 grams, just under 2 pounds, she had suffered through almost three weeks of severe respiratory distress. Her physical condition had improved markedly in the past week, Hannan noted, but she still had overwhelming "social problems." As best the nurses and the hospital's social service department could piece things together, Darleeta's mother had been or still was a drug addict. She apparently had a deep distrust of social workers and anyone else (like the nurses and physicians at Metropolitan) whom she viewed as authority figures. Not only hadn't the infant's mother come to visit her, but also only one of the nurses, a young woman on the evening shift named Beth Lockridge, had ever managed to contact Darleeta's mother by telephone. Beth had talked to the woman three times in the four weeks the baby had been in the nursery but had had no luck convincing her to come in to visit her child.

Socially, Stephen Durand was Darleeta Smith's opposite. In his four years at Metropolitan, Jim Hannan had never come across another couple quite like Robert and Jessica Durand. He had seen devotion before; most of the parents cared about their sick babies. And there had been other couples who had spent hours at a time in the nursery, with its unlimited access for parents. But the Durands were the extreme. It seemed to Hannan that one or both of the baby's parents were always in the nursery, twenty-four hours a day. At least Hannan was sure he had never walked into the nursery when Stephen was there and not seen at least one of the baby's parents.

Born thirty-five days earlier weighing 1,180 grams (2.6 pounds), Stephen Durand now weighed only 1,110 grams. He had finally come off the respirator after a protracted siege with respiratory distress syndrome (RDS) and had now apparently developed bronchopulmonary dysplasia. Like several of the other babies in the nursery this Christmas Eve, he had had sepsis, and in addition he had had a collapsed lung. From what Hannan could tell from initial X-rays, Stephen Durand was functioning on approximately a quarter of his lungs' total volume. But he had certainly looked better when Hannan left town Tuesday than he had a few days before that.

As Hannan was preparing to flip the cardex shut, his eyes came to rest on Cato Adams' card. Born by cesarean section thirteen days earlier, Cato, at 1,500 grams, had been small for his gestational age, or at least what his mother's obstetrician thought the infant's gestational age was. But he had already gained 70 grams and appeared to be doing well. He suffered from hypospadius, a malformation of the penis that could be surgically corrected when he was older. Hannan often wondered what the statistics on these premies would be if the statisticians stuck to counting congenital malformations and defects that weren't correctable, and that would prevent the baby from leading a normal life, rather than counting every harelip, cleft palate, and malformed . . . "Oh, what the hell," he thought, slamming shut the aluminum covers of the cardex, "let's get this show on the road."

Rising from his chair, Hannan shoved a meticulously sharpened yellow pencil into the thick brown hair falling over his left ear. He neglected to notice that he already had a similar pencil protruding from behind his right ear. Pushing his hair back out of his eyes, he took the short-sleeved nursery gown that hung on one of the hooks on the back of his office door, pulled it on, opened the door, and stepped into Rita Andrews' "office."

"I'll be in the nursery, Rita. By the way, have you finished typing that stuff I gave you for Perinatal Press?"

"Not yet, Dr. Hannan."

"Okay. But see if you can get it done before you leave tonight. I really need to get that out. Thanks," he added, as he headed down the hall to the nursery, his hands busy tying the back of his gown shut.

Chapter Three

The Intensive Care Nursery at Metropolitan Lying-In Hospital is divided into three main rooms, with two 7½ × 12 foot entrance areas separating Rooms A, B, and C. The first of these areas, dividing Rooms B and C, is the entrance used by visitors to the nursery or by staff members who have been out of the nursery area and need to scrub up again. It is also the entrance closest to Jim Hannan's office, and as he entered the nursery for daily rounds he stepped up to the sink immediately to the left of the door and followed the instructions posted there, not that he needed to read the reminder to:

"1—Remove watch and all rings except plain wedding band.

"2—Scrub fingernails.

"3—Wash hands and arms to elbows for a full three minutes.

"4—Wear cover gown tied in back (long-sleeved gown if you are wearing long sleeves.)"

Standing at the sink, Hannan could look over his left shoulder through a picture window into the "putrid pink" C room, the high-risk area of the nursery, where three babies lay bundled in open, clear lucite cribs, much as they would be in the regular nurseries downstairs. Despite the fact that there were only three babies in the 13 × 14 foot area, it was as cramped as the rest of the nursery, a barely organized jumble of spare Isolettes, a portable infant X-ray unit, two spare respirators (one if you didn't count the transport respirator, which Hannan would rather not have to count as one of his seven ventilators), a scale for weighing the babies, and two white rocking chairs for the use of nurses and mothers feeding their infants. The entry room, too, was crowded, taken up as it was by the stainless-steel sink at which Hannan stood, the nursery's air compressor, a table for working on charts and records, and a counter and supply cabinets with glass doors along the wall opposite the sink.

To Hannan's right, also visible through a plate-glass window, lay Room B, one of the two main rooms in the nursery. On this day there were four Isolettes and two warming tables, one of them in use, in the 16 × 19 foot area. The green walls were a less institutional color than the mauve of Room C, but they certainly weren't a color a parent would be likely to pick for a baby's room. An X-ray light box was mounted on the exterior end wall, next to the double windows that framed a glorious view of the hospital's back parking lot. The set of chest X-rays left on the light box served as a reminder of the type of patient served by the nursery: the entire chest and abdomen displayed on the negative film were smaller than a good-sized adult hand. One of the nurses had hung a sentimental woodland scene above the light box, bearing the words, "The greatest thing a father can do for his children is love their mother." The opposite wall was dominated by a set of double picture windows that afforded parents and other visitors in the hallway a view of this area of the nursery. One of the Isolettes was pushed up against that wall, while a second stood against the opposite wall, under the windows. A third Isolette and the warming table on which baby Fisher lay, were standing along the long wall nearest the entrance room and Jim Hannan, while another Isolette and Becky Fontain's warming table took up the space on the other side of the room. What area there was in the middle of the room was taken up by another of the nursery's white rockers and a steady flow of human traffic moving back and forth among the Isolettes and warming tables.

"Merry Christmas, Dr. Hannan," chirped Pat Ward, one of the newer day-shift nurses, as she stepped into the entrance area to peel off a blood-spattered cover gown.

"Hi, Pat," said Hannan, looking up from inspecting his immaculate nails. "Have special plans for tomorrow?"

"I'm on during the day," answered the twenty-two-year-old woman as she shoved the soiled gown into the large plastic-bag-lined laundry hamper near the sink, "but I'm going to my boyfriend's parents' place for Christmas dinner after I get off."

"Well, have a nice time, if I don't see you again," said Hannan.

"I'm sure you will," said the nurse, walking out into the hallway. Jim Hannan finished drying his hands with a paper towel from the dispenser over the sink, picked up his cardex, and headed into the main nursery, where his entrance always affected the staff, particularly the nurses, much as an approaching summer thunderstorm touches off some sixth sense in animals miles away: There would be an almost imperceptible stiffening of backs, a checking of small details, a quick look to make sure monitor alarms hadn't been turned off, a search for psychic shelter from the usually quiet but usually deeply biting remarks that would follow the discovery of some minute error or slip-up.

"Ready, Ravi?" Hannan asked Javed, who was writing medication orders for baby McKnight in the nursery office area between Rooms A and B.

"I'll be with you in just one minute," replied Javed, glancing up. But Hannan, whose question had been a summons, hadn't stopped to hear the answer and had already passed through the area, into Room A.

The A room, 445, was even more chaotic-looking than the

back room with all its spare equipment. Here lay the majority of the ICN's patients, eight in Isolettes and two on warming tables. The room was designed as an open area, but the Isolettes running along the walls and protruding from one of the walls at angles formed bays in which the nurses and physicians worked. One of the long walls was taken up with a sink for hand washing, the door to the hallway, a counter where the baby scale was kept and where the ICN's hand calculator was literally chained down, and storage areas for other small bits of equipment. The opposite and end walls were lined with babies and equipment. A giant stick-on decal of a pink hippopotamus watched over the babies from one wall, while a giraffe decal peered over baby McKnight's warming table against the end wall. To the nurses' eternal credit, the "Hang in There Baby" poster showing a kitten dangling by its forepaws (a poster found in some size or version in most Intensive Care Nurseries) was mercifully absent from the walls of Metropolitan's ICN.

By the time Javed caught up with Jim Hannan, rounds had already begun. The senior man had used baby Durand's case as the basis for a discussion of bronchopulmonary dysplasia. Hannan was speaking quietly as Javed approached, for, true to form, Robert Durand was in the nursery visiting his son. Immobile as the Isolette in which his son lay, Durand sat staring at the sleeping infant.

The group of physicians and medical students stood in a tight semicircle, with Hannan in the center, making notes in his cardex. Each of the other men and women in the group held either a small, overflowing notebook or a loose stack of 3 × 5 cards to which they referred when called upon, or which they used to take notes. Some, like medical student Martin Wells, nervously fingered the cards, bending their edges and worrying them with their hands. They dreaded being called upon but, at the same time, hoped for a chance to impress Hannan with a bit of knowledge he might not have expected them to pick up.

"Does anybody know what vitamin E does?" Hannan asked as Javed joined the group.

"It's an antioxident," responded Wells, his reply more a question than a statement.

"Ah, that's right," said Hannan, looking directly at Wells, "but that's not going to get you any points. How does it act as an antioxident?" Wells' eyes were downcast, staring at the cards whose edges he was busily tattering with his long fingers. "Does anybody know?" Hannan asked. Silence. "Why don't you all join hands," he told the puzzled group. "Over on this end, in your right hand," he said to Karen Fitzgerald, a first-year pediatric resident from St. Francis, "there's a sort of hydrophilic tail. Then there's a long train of double-bonded carbon atoms that string out like that," he said, running his hands along the line formed by the joined hands of Karen Fitzgerald, Wells, medical student Saul Goodman, and Fellow John Noble. "The oxygen in the lungs comes by and sits on a double bond like this and it gets converted into electrons, which then take off, and it doesn't do a whole lot for bonding. So here is this vitamin E. It sits right in the membrane," he said, pointing to the spaces where each set of hands joined. "You can let go now, unless you get off on that." The students laughed. "I want you to remember this because the vitamin E sits in the interstices of the lipid membrane and it doesn't act as a vitamin; it acts as a metabolite. It gets eaten up by oxygen to a certain extent, but it gets eaten up instead of the membrane itself. And that's why you give milligrams of vitamin E, instead of the micrograms we give of other vitamins. You give a little baby 50 to 100 milligrams of vitamin E under normal circumstances and he's got enough vitamin E there to keep him fertile for the next three eons, right? A baby doesn't need much vitamin E in terms of its fertility effect or its effect on hair growth. But in terms of its protective effect, a baby needs a lot of E in order to get it into all these developing lipid membranes and actually act as a sort of mechanical shield. You ever watch 'Star Trek' on TV?" he asked Fitzgerald.

"Yes, but why?" she asked, wondering how the discussion had shifted in a breath from lipid membranes and BPD to Captain James Kirk and the crew of the Starship Enterprise.

"Because they put up these shields to protect against laser beams. Well, look what vitamin E does for the membrane: It lays out in the membrane itself, and then the oxygen can't do the membrane in." While Hannan's explanation may have seemed overly complex to the third-year students, stressing the molecular basis of the treatment rather than treatment schedules or known effectiveness, the tack he took was carefully calculated, based as it was on his belief that it is impossible to treat a patient without thoroughly understanding the science behind the treatment. If a physician doesn't have total knowledge of why a particular drug or form of therapy works under certain circumstances, Hannan felt, he couldn't hope to understand why it failed to work in a given case. And such a failure of understanding could lead directly to the death of a patient. Thus he wanted the students and Fellows not only to understand that vitamin E seems to play a role in preventing the stiffening of the lung associated with BPD, but also to understand why it acts as it does.

Before listening to Saul Goodman's presentation of baby Greene's case, Hannan asked Javed whether the infant's parents had agreed, while Hannan was gone, to have Andrew placed on an experimental protocol for the treatment of a thyroid condition from which he suffered. Andrew himself lay on a warming table, across the aisle from baby Durand. At 6½ pounds, he looked totally out of place among the other infants who resembled frying chickens more than full-term babies. But the constant "Eeet! eeet! eeet! eeet! eeet!" of his heart monitor, the rhythmic wheezing of his respirator, and the tan blinders protecting his eyes from the ultraviolet lights being used to treat his moderate jaundice left no doubt that he belonged where he was.

"The parents didn't want him in the study," Javed explained to Hannan, "but they wanted to know if he could get the drug anyway. I told them I would talk to you and we might be able . . ."

"Wait a minute," interjected Hannan. "Are you familiar with what a double-blind study's all about?" He was leaning forward from the waist, his face jutting out toward Javed, his twin yellow pencils pointing forward threateningly, like the horns of an irritated bull. "If a parent enrolls in the study, you tell them that the effects are not known, although we think they're beneficial, and that the side effects are not known either. And the gamble is essentially that we're using a drug and watching for side effects, or not using a drug and watching for lack of effect, and there's no way of knowing which. If you know which baby is receiving the drug and which is receiving the placebo, that's not a double-blind study. If the parents choose not to go into the study," Hannan told the group, and Javed in particular, "then you've got the problem of saying, 'What do you do? Do you treat or don't you treat?' Now with Greene, the parents have said they don't want the kid in the study, so the kid's not getting the drug. Now if they change their minds and want us to use the drug, I can't in good conscience say whether he should or shouldn't get it. They have to make a decision and then we have to agree with it. Some investigators say, 'If the kid doesn't improve in two weeks, then we'll assume he's on the placebo and give him the drug.' But that's not a double-blind study. That's not a valid experimental design: That's a cop-out," declared Hannan, clearly disgusted with the idea of such investigative game playing.

"It's not a double-blind study?" asked Javed.

"Not unless it's designed as a crossover," Hannan continued, "a part of the study to break the double-blind at two weeks. But then you've got to do the same thing for everybody in the study. But if you simply do it because there's no effect on the kid, then you're basing your research on the premise that your hypothesis about the drug is correct. If you're assuming that, then you have no right to do a study. Either test your hypothesis with an open mind or let someone else, who isn't biased, test it.

"I know Rich has some reservations about whether the study should be done," said Hannan, referring to Dr. Richard Sherrill, another of the unit's three fully trained neonatologists. "He thinks it's perfectly reasonable to use thyroid. I thought it was reasonable to use it in the past, because we didn't have a study going, so we used it. But I feel there's enough of a testable hypothesis so we should be doing this study. It's my study, and switching a kid over to the drug if he isn't getting well isn't part of the study design. So it's not an option. Parents can stop the study. They can say, 'I don't want my baby to get the drug anymore.' They can leave the study. But that's an action independent of the study. Or they can say, 'I don't want you to give the drug,' like this kid's parents did. That's just like somebody refusing penicillin or blood. Then you have to make some other decisions about treatment. But they can't say, 'I want you to stop the study and give the drug,' because that means that their judgment about whether the drug should be used is more correct than yours."

"But what if a parent changes her mind? What if she thinks better of an earlier decision that she didn't want to risk having her baby in a study?" John Noble asked.

"Look, you just don't do research that way. They have all the options laid out at the beginning and that's when they have to make their decision." Hannan was clearly getting irritated that even the Fellows, who had completed four years of pre-med, four years of medical school, and at least three years of pediatric residency and were now in subspecialty training, failed to grasp such basic principles of research design. "This may seem like a subtle point, but it's a problem a lot of people in research have: They assume, in various ways, that their hypothesis is correct, and they link their test system with cop-outs to prove the hypothesis. What would you do if you give the drug to every baby and they all improve? You don't know how long to give the drug or when to give it. You have no data. Just remember this: There are two ways to do research; a right way and a wrong way.

"I call your attention to a book you were given, and I suggested you read," Hannan told the group, "called *Research and Design.* It talks about fourteen different methodological approaches to research. It'll show you how to do a patient crossover, if that's what you want. If you really wanted to test that hypothesis, you could say 'I'll take all the kids with a low thyroid level, I'll give them all either the placebo or the real drug, and then, at two-week intervals, I'll switch them over.' That's a legitimate strategy. But there's a major problem you run into with that in neonatal medicine," Hannan reminded them, "where that strategy doesn't work: The baby as an organism is going to change. It's going to grow and mature. So that when you do the study over a two- or four-week period of time, you're really not doing it on the same patient; you're doing it on a two- or four-week older patient. You've got to decide what you're going to do, do it with each baby at the same stage, and then follow it. If you say 'I'm going to test the hypothesis and then if the hypothesis doesn't work out in four days I'm going to give the drug,' that doesn't make any sense! It's not rational! It's not logical! And we hope one does research on a rational basis. If not, you say, 'Well, in my experience I did such and such and it worked,' and God knows the world doesn't need any more papers like that. But enough. Let's move on. Who's next?"

"Baby Fisher," said Martin Wells.

"Okay, what about him?"

"He's a twenty-eight-week gestation, 740 grams, present weight of 1,060, which is an increase of 30 over yesterday. Do you want me to go over the history?"

"No," Hannan snapped sarcastically, "I don't want to spend more than four hours on rounds." He knew full well that on the mornings following his return to nursery duty, whether he had been away three days or three weeks, rounds seemed to take at least two hours.

"Okay. He's presently a Silverman of 3," said Wells, referring to a system for scoring a baby's difficulty in breathing, a Silverman of zero being the best score and 10 the worst, "on an IMV of 2, when last I checked, Peak of 19."

"If he's on this machine you can't do IMV," said Hannan,

34

pointing to the Bourns pressure respirator. "Now, why is he not on a volume ventilator instead of this pressure machine? Don't we have any volume ventilators?"

"We can do IMV on this . . ." began Javed.

"You can't do IMV on this ventilator," Hannan cut Javed off.

Javed tried again to persuade Hannan that a baby could be given the treatment Hannan thought appropriate on the pressure ventilator, but to no avail.

"You can't do IMV on this ventilator! Why can't you do IMV on this ventilator? What does IMV stand for?" he demanded of the Fellow.

"Intermittent mandatory ventilation," Javed answered. The machine forces the infant to take a certain number of breaths per minute, at chosen intervals, no matter what the infant does on his own.

"Right. Ventilation. Now, what makes up ventilation? Volume of gas times number of breaths per minute. What's the volume he's receiving? You don't know! You can make some assumptions, but in a kid who's got crap in his lungs and changing compliance [changing "give" or ability to expand in the lung] and changing delivery of volume, you can't do it. Even with this *on!*" He angrily reached over and switched on the respirator alarm, which responded with an angry "Eeeeeeeeee!" One of the little details sure to set Hannan off was finding an alarm switch turned to "off," so that a light blinked—but no alarm sounded—if there was a problem. Because the constant scream of the alarms would begin to drive them a bit daffy, the nurses would often turn off the alarm when an infant kept triggering it by moving around. But Hannan believed the alarms were an integral part of the equipment. There was no point in monitoring an infant if you didn't know when something was going wrong.

The dispute over the volume versus the pressure ventilator centered on the basic function of the two types of respirators. The pressure respirator is designed to deliver a mixture of gases, at a preselected pressure and with a certain force, to the infant's lungs. The volume ventilator, however, delivers a preselected volume, or amount, of gas to the lungs. In order to make sure an infant is moving the proper amount of gas—oxygen in and carbon dioxide out—with each breath, it is essential to control the volume of gas he receives, rather than the pressure at which the gas is delivered.

"I don't understand," Hannan told the group. "This kid should never have come off a volume ventilator. Was he on and then taken off? Is that what happened?"

"No, he was never on," Karen Fitzgerald told him. "There was nothing available. At the time, Odell was on a volume ventilator, Scott was on a volume ventilator, Durand was on one, and there was nothing left."

"Do we only have three volume ventilators?"

"Well," Fitzgerald tried to explain, "there's the old Bourns, but they decided against putting him on that."

"This is suboptimal," Hannan told her, clearly not satisfied with the explanation. "Now, why did he go back on the ventilator in the first place? He had come off."

"He had bradycardia and apnea [periods of decreased heart rate and cessation of breathing]," Wells told him.

"When was this?"

"Day before yesterday," Javed told his boss.

"What was the cause of the apnea and bradycardia? CO_2 retention?"

"There was some question of sepsis at the time," said Martin Wells, "and some of the bradycardia appeared to be caused by suctioning [secretions from the lungs]."

"What made you think there was a question of sepsis?" Hannan asked.

"I wasn't there at that time," Wells began to explain, but Hannan cut him short, demanding of Javed, "You were here, right? So you should know."

"The cultures grew strep," Javed told him.

"Strep what?"

"Um, strep, um," he stumbled, unsure of the answer without consulting the chart.

"Strep B?"

"That was it."

"So he was put on penicillin?" Hannan asked.

"Yea."

"Just penicillin?"

"Just penicillin initially," Javed explained, "but then the baby had bradycardia and apnea and they suspected sepsis, so they put him on kanamycin."

"What was his spinal tap? It was negative?"

"It was negative," said Wells. "No cultures, the cultures were negative."

"So that was the reason he was put on the ventilator, because he had bradycardia and apnea? Did he have any CO_2 retention?"

"Not today," said Wells, checking the chart lying on the warming table beside the shallow plexiglass pan in which the baby lay.

"What's his aminophyllin level?" Hannan asked Wells.

"Six."

"Okay. I would suggest you put him on a volume ventilator, the same IMV, and give him about a half-second hold. Try to get his lungs cleared, because they sound lousy," Hannan said as he leaned over the tiny baby, listening to his chest with a stethoscope. He stood back up, laying the stethoscope on the silver-gray warming table. "Evie, what are you getting out of his lungs? A lot of crap?"

"Yeah," replied Evie Roth, Sam Fisher's primary nurse. Each baby in the nursery had a primary nurse—one person responsible for writing nursing orders and overseeing nursing care. Even though the primary nurse is only on one eight-hour shift in a twenty-four-hour day, the system also guarantees some continuity of nursing care and assures the parents that one person knows what's happening to their baby on a minute-by-minute basis.

Like the other ICN nurses, Evie's day revolved around the

one or two babies in her charge. Because Sam Fisher was on a respirator, he was receiving one-to-one nursing care—he was Evie's sole responsibility. While she would help out with other babies when she had a free minute, Sam always came first. Unlike the unit nurse in a general hospital, the twenty-four-year-old woman spent all but her lunch hour within about 10 feet of her patient, and most of the eight-hour shift she was beside his warming table suctioning secretions from his lungs and throat, responding to monitor alarms, changing diapers the size of tiny sanitary napkins, sterilizing equipment for future use, and administering medications through Sam's IVs. To some, the minute baby lying on the table might have looked more like a newborn monkey than a human baby, and the analogy was an apt one, for at 2.3 pounds Sam Fisher looked nothing like the baby on the Gerber jar. His light brown skin was translucent, revealing all his surface veins and the outlines of all his matchstick-like ribs. His flat little nose protruded from the oversize blinders protecting his eyes from the ultraviolet light that was breaking down his bilirubin. When he moved his arms and legs, none of which was longer than Evie Roth's hand, he moved them in a choppy, almost mechanical fashion. But to the nurse, as well as to his mother, Sam Fisher was a beautiful little baby, a baby in whom they could already see an emerging personality as he responded to handling and to the pain of IVs and the other equipment that engulfed him.

Continuing with his comments, Hannan noted that the "crap" which Evie was removing from the baby's lungs was his problem. "See, they get secretions that occlude their tubes and then they get bradycardias because they're hypoxic. There's nothing magical; it's just like if I grabbed you by the throat," he told Wells; "you'd get hypoxic too. You've just got to suction 'em out. I know logistics are a problem, but that's when you get caught off base. That's when you've got to lean on the respiratory therapy department. You can't handle this kid on this ventilator. So get respiratory therapy up here, get 'em to supply the ventilator you

need, get 'em to clean it. If you've got problems getting the
ventilator sterilized, make sure they do it. If you have any further problems," he told the medical students and resident, "call
the attending physician on duty and he'll call the administrator.
You don't build a house with a sledge hammer," he summed up,
"and that's what you were trying to do by putting this baby on a
pressure respirator. This just isn't the right tool for this kid.
Okay, so that's his ventilatory status. What else?"

"Other than that, we just got his bilirubin back. It's 11.7."

"Why?" Hannan demanded, knowing that the baby's bilirubin
had been much lower when Hannan left town three days ago.
Bilirubin, a yellowish pigment in the bile, is broken down in the
liver in the mature, healthy human system. But in many premature babies, and in some full-term newborns, the liver is unable
to break down the chemical and jaundice results. When that
happens, ultraviolet light can be used to break down the chemical by causing photooxidation in the skin. Baby Fisher, his eyes
protected by cloth blinders, was lying under the ultraviolet
lights.

"Oh, wait a minute!" exclaimed Wells, rechecking his tattered
note cards. "That's baby Lincoln's bili! Fisher's is fine." The
discussion continued as Wells presented the baby's nutritional
status and then returned to the question of his possible sepsis and
the antibiotics.

"The cultures were negative, right?" Hannan asked John Noble, who nodded affirmatively. "Then I would have taken him off
the antibiotics when the cultures came back. How long was he
on?"

"Seven days," Noble told him.

"That's a long time to get a culture back."

"The culture came back before that," said Noble, who usually
had the right answers for Hannan but now was clearly on a
collision course with his boss.

"Then you should have stopped the antibiotics when you got
the negative cultures back. This is something you and I will have
to get to know about each other," Hannan told the younger

physician. "I think you need some strong evidence, meaning positive cultures, to continue antibiotics. I have no objections, if you think a baby's clinically septic, to start with what you think are appropriate antibiotics while you get the tests and so forth. Then you have to set up criteria in your mind for when you will establish the diagnosis of sepsis. When those criteria aren't met, then you've got to stop the use of antibiotics. It's not rational to continue. You've got to remember that sepsis can be caused by virus, which the antibiotics won't touch, as well as by bacteria. So you and I will be having a lot of jumping up and down and screaming and yelling if I hear a lot of kids get treated for suspected sepsis and they're continued on antibiotics for ten or eleven days in the face of negative cultures."

"But a negative culture doesn't rule out sepsis," Noble argued.

"Look," Hannan said firmly, "you've really got to stop and think about this. You can ask yourself with any baby that comes through the door, 'Could this baby possibly be septic?' And the answer's yes. Well, okay, cultures don't rule out sepsis. So you might as well start putting antibiotics in the drinking water. What I'm saying to you is that you've got to set up criteria. You've got to say to yourself, 'I think this baby's septic. Why? Well, he's got a temperature, apnea, and bradycardia, clinical signs. Okay, now, how am I going to prove it? Well, I'm going to do some CBCs and cultures and so forth, and I'm going to set up some specific clinical criteria that will worry me.' Now! If those criteria aren't met, you've *got* to stop the antibiotics. If the kid's sed rate goes up, you start antibiotics. If the kid's sed rate goes down, he stops having apnea and bradycardia, he looks a lot better, and the cultures come back negative. *Then,* by objective measurement, you're in a little better position to argue with me that the kid was septic but the cultures didn't reflect it.

"But all you tell me about this kid," Hannan continued, gesturing toward baby Fisher, "is that he had apnea and bradycardia and had his aminophyllin increased. All this means is that you sterilized his trachea 'cause it didn't grow strep anymore, and he had a negative blood culture. First, that suggests he shouldn't have been put on kanamycin, and *certainly* kanamycin shouldn't have been continued when you found out everything was negative. *And,* whatever the reasons for them, the symptoms disappeared much too quickly for the antibiotics to be making the difference, so I think you probably should have stopped the antibiotics after three days. *Now,* the only way you're going to be able to argue with me rationally is if you set those data up, because then it's your opinion versus mine and your opinion's just as good as mine. If you've got the facts, it's better than mine. Otherwise, we're gonna have arguments all the time. And remember, if he is septic, you've got to continue the antibiotics for ten days to two weeks. If you don't have hard facts, you're going to fall into this middle ground, and it's an irrational position. You'll end up with the same problem as everywhere: *Everybody* gets put on antibiotics. Everybody gets a mild set first, then after twelve, eighteen days they get a stronger medication. I'm just trying to keep you from getting into a hole, because I'm waiting at the bottom," concluded Hannan with an evil grin. "Okay, what else have we got?"

"We just got his blood volume, hematocrits and . . ." began Wells.

"Tell me about his 'electric lights' first," interjected Hannan, making a pun of electrolytes, the chemicals whose balance controls all the body's electrical activity, including that of the heart and central nervous system.

"His electrolytes haven't come back yet this morning, but they've been normal," Wells told him.

"Okay, tell me about his blood volume status. What an interesting term," he added, drawing a laugh from most of group.

"Well, his perfusion is good. He had 12 ccs transfused back in last night so now his hematocrit's back up."

"Can you tell me anything more about his intravascular compartment I might want to know?"

"Not much," Wells admitted. "We're waiting for a total protein."

"That's part of my standing order, isn't it? The lab's supposed to do a total protein and hematocrit on every baby once a week."

"They're doing the new babies twice a week," Javed told him, as though the fact that the new babies were being checked twice as often as required was sufficient explanation for the older infants' not being checked as often as required.

"Well, they're supposed to be doing every baby in here once a week. I'll have to talk to Jesus," said Hannan, referring to Jesus Ortega, the director of the ICN's lab, located two doors down the hall from the nursery. "Where's a card?" Hannan asked himself aloud, searching through his cardex. Saul Goodman handed him a blank 3 × 5 card. "Thanks. Talk to Jesus," Hannan said, writing it with one of the yellow pencils. "Okay. Who's next?"

And so they worked their way through the nursery, stopping at each baby long enough for one of the junior staff members or trainees to give a complete presentation of the baby's present metabolic and overall status, including any changes in condition since the last rounds. Because Hannan had been away for three days, and perhaps because some of the group's thoughts seemed to be on the upcoming holiday as much as on the charts, the going was slow. It was also painful for the medical students or residents who had failed to pay attention on earlier rounds, as appeared to be the case during Karen Fitzgerald's presentation of baby Odell.

"The child had respiratory distress at delivery, had to be intubated, and then was brought upstairs. Since that time . . ."

"Why was the baby intubated?" Hannan demanded, knowing the answer just as he knew the answers to virtually all his other questions.

"Because the baby was not breathing," Fitzgerald told him.

"Why was not the baby breathing?"

"Because it was unable to breathe on its own, probably due to prematurity."

"You believe that?" Hannan asked, sarcastically. "Anybody who believes that, raise their hands."

"I believe it," Fitzgerald said in a near whisper.

"That prematures don't breath because they're immature?"

"No, because of immaturity of the lungs and surfactant."

"Ah, immaturity of the lungs and lung surfactant," Hannan mused, tugging at his thin mustache with his lower lip and acting as though Fitzgerald was telling him something new.

"Lack of surfactant," corrected Fitzgerald.

"Say he had decreased surfactant, what would that do to his respiration?"

"It would . . ."

"What is the hallmark of idiopathic respiratory distress syndrome?" Hannan asked, verbally climbing all over Fitzgerald.

"Gasping?"

"No! Wrong! PLEASE READ the section in Klaus and Fanaroff on hyaline membrane disease, respiratory distress, again. Do you know?" he asked, turning to Martin Wells.

"Nasal flaring, retractions, cyanosis," which is blue coloration caused by a lack of oxygen.

"What is the hallmark of respiratory distress for whatever cause? Suppose I grabbed her by the throat?" He placed his hands around Fitzgerald's throat, causing her to jump back.

"Gasping?" guessed Wells.

"She breathes fast! She breathes fast! She gets tachypnea [rapid breathing]. Kids with hyaline membrane disease get tachypnea," he said, stressing every word by rhythmically hitting the wall with his fist. "They get hypoxic, they get acidotic and all the other unpleasantness, and then they get apnic and bradycardic. Okay? Hyaline membrane disease kids get breathing fast. Now, let's go back. This kid wasn't breathing at birth?"

"He was breathing at birth," Fitzgerald told him, changing what she had said earlier.

"He was breathing. Then why did he get intubated?" he asked, referring to the little girl by the masculine pronoun, a mistake most of the physicians, male or female, made with amazing frequency.

"He stopped breathing."

"He stopped breathing. Ah ha! Why did he stop breathing? You say it's not because his lungs were massively collapsed. He got hypoxic. Why did he get hypoxic?"

"Because segments of his lungs were not able to open up and get ventilated," said Fitzgerald.

"I would argue that would be very unusual," Hannan said, "unless he had something in there, like pneumonia. Are there any other reasons to explain why he stopped breathing? I'm trying to get you to understand that prematurity per se is not a cause of asphyxia at birth. Prematurity is frequently statistically associated with asphyxia at birth, but if you look at it as a cause, it's only going to lead you down a blind alley. As a matter of fact, that's one of the reasons why, in the District of Columbia, everybody says that neonatal mortality is due to unexplained immaturity. The level of thinking has stopped at that point. Too bad for the District of Columbia. Now, do you know of any other reasons that can cause kids to be asphyxiated? Do we know what medications his mother was given during her travail to deliver this poor unfortunate?"

"Well, the mother was given an alcohol IV drip during the day to delay labor," Fitzgerald told him, checking her notes.

"Oh, Lord! What does alcohol do to your breathing?" Hannan asked in mock shock.

"Well, it'll cause depression," said Fitzgerald.

"What's that called?"

"Respiratory depression?" replied the young woman, reaching for an answer to please him and end her humiliation.

"It's called dead drunk. These babies can get dead drunk. How does alcohol cause depressed respiration?"

"It has a direct effect on the respiratory center of the brain."

"Ah, and what do we say about the respiratory centers of these babies? They're immature. They don't do their thing in the same way as yours and mine, unless we have a five-martini lunch."

After wrapping up the discussion of baby Odell's respiratory problems, the group moved along to Darleeta Smith. "We're really having problems with the social situation here," Saul Goodman told Hannan. "None of us has succeeded in contacting the mother. We know that Beth has talked to her a few times, but that hasn't been much help to us. We need more information about the pregnancy and the mother's condition, and we're also worried about where she's going when she leaves here. Is this a case for protective services?"

"If you want that kind of information, then you have to write a social services consult. Let's see, you say Beth's the primary nurse and she's evenings? I've requested that if we as physicians want social services to get involved (and that's independently of the nursing staff), we ought to write specific questions to get them answered. Otherwise we get amorphous garbage, and everybody just sits down and holds hands and acts friendly. I think you can use social services very profitably because they have great skill in getting this kind of information, but you have to ask the right questions. Specifically: Given the social circumstances of this lady, what are her psychological supports? Her husband? Is there a husband? Her mother? Where is she going to be living? Also, if you feel there are some specific emotional or psychological problems, you might get a consult with a psychiatrist. Everything else that social services wants to do for this mother is fine, but if we want the answers to specific questions, then we have to ask them, and we have to have them answered in such a way that everybody who's responsible for this kid's care when you and I aren't here knows about them. Okay?"

When the group came to baby Fontain, in the B room, Javed skimmed over Becky's ninety days in the nursery, speaking quietly out of deference to Charlotte Fontain, who stood by the warming table. She was gently stroking her daughter's tiny naked leg and staring off into space. Javed explained that various formulas and feeding methods had been tried, but to no avail. Nothing had succeeded in putting weight on the baby. After listening to Javed for almost twenty minutes and asking almost forty questions in that time, Hannan said, "I thought we agreed before I left to get her transferred to St. Francis?"

"We've been calling every day," explained Javed, "but they say either they haven't got the space, or they don't have anybody to pick her up."

"Well then, we'll take her over, and we're going to do it today. This crap has got to stop," said Hannan. "Look, troops, here's my hypothesis," he said, beginning an explanation of the need to transfer the baby. "We've gone the whole nine yards with this baby. We've done an upper (GI series) and flipped the kid over and what we seem to have here is an obstructive pattern. One way or another, somewhere up high in this kid's GI tract, there's got to be an obstruction. Okay? There's no way around it. We keep putting food in there and no matter what it is, whether it's water with some sugar in it, or formula, it don't go through. So what has to happen now is that she has to have a little more evaluation and she has to have her belly cracked. What we've got to do is convince Bob Albert [a pediatric surgeon] to take her over to that great bastion of neonatal referral, St. Francis, and do it. He needs to have somebody look in there with a fiberoptic-scope, and there probably isn't anyone there with enough skill and a scope small enough to know what they're looking at. They need to do another barium series, probably, to know what's going on, and then they need to explore this baby."

"It's been ninety days and this baby has not been feeding nearly enough. But I thought some barium did go through when we had it done earlier, so I don't know if there's an obstruction," said Javed, disagreeing with Hannan's analysis.

"That's like saying a 'little ulcer,' or a 'little tumor,' or a 'little whatever-you've-got,' " countered Hannan. "The point is this baby has enough obstruction to interfere with normal absorption of nutrition. Aside from that, you've had to nourish this kid in a way that is fraught with its own problems. You've got a process and a complication of the management of the process. I'm all for the medical, rather than the surgical, management of various diseases, even when we don't know what the diseases are. But I think we've gotten past that point with this particular baby. We've gotten the baby in fairly good metabolic shape; at least it's better than it was—she isn't starving. Well, I think we've messed around long enough. And I don't say that critically. I think she's had all the trials of a variety of things and I think we've reached the point, quite frankly, where we don't have a whole lot more to offer her. So get hold of Bob Albert and have him give me a call. Okay?"

"Charlotte," he began, stepping over to Becky's mother, who, after three months, was on a first-name basis with many of the nursery staffers, "I want to appologize for the fact that it's taken so long to set up this transfer. Dr. Noble tells me you've taken the last three days off from work, and I'm really sorry things have gotten so messed up. We'll try to get them straightened out and have her over there by this evening. Do you have any new questions? I know we've talked several times about the transfer."

"No. I understand everything," said Charlotte Fontain, looking up at Hannan. Her large, deep, brown eyes told of every minute, hour, day, week, and month she had sat at the warming table watching her daughter fail to live, if not die. "I know you're doing what you can." She reached out and touched Hannan's hand, which was resting on the warming table.

"Thank you," he said quietly. "I'll be talking to you again before we move her. All right," he said, more brusquely, turning back to the physicians, "who's next?"

"Baby Breslin," Javed told him.

"Oh, the one the mother doesn't want," said Hannan, laughing as Catherine Breslin, who was sitting two feet away rocking her baby, playfully kicked at Hannan's shins. Even though Susie Breslin now weighed just over four pounds, she looked like a field mouse as her six-foot-tall mother held her in her lap. "Howdy," said Hannan, "how you doing?"

"Okay," replied a smiling Catherine Breslin.

"Pretty soon she won't be on our service," Hannan told her.

"Susie's up to 1,840 grams," said Javed.

"Terrific!" Hannan told the baby's mother, his warmth and openness with her, as it had been with Charlotte Fontain, a direct contrast to his manner with the group on rounds. "Any questions?" he asked the mother.

"No. You're all doing a terrific job. I couldn't be happier," she said, beaming at the baby, who lay in her lap wearing a stocking cap embroidered by a proud grandmother with "Harvard 2001." All the babies looked unbelievably small lying in an adult's arms, but the contrast between Susie Breslin and her mother struck the staff as particularly amusing, perhaps because it was common to see a six-foot father whose hands covered the greater part of his infant's body, but a six-foot mother was another matter. But little Susie had reached the point where she would smile slightly in response to her mother's coooing and laughing conversation, at times seeming to almost grin as the huge adult face loomed down over her.

"All right, gang, that's it for today. If I don't see you all later, Merry Christmas. But I'm sure I will. See you." Hannan and most of those on rounds laughed.

"Have you got a minute, Jim?" asked John Noble.

"Not right now. I've got to get down to education rounds." Hannan walked out of the nursery, throwing his gown in the laundry bin in the entrance room. As the door closed behind Hannan, Martin Wells, who was talking to the remaining members of the group, dropped to his knees and clasped his hands in a mock prayer of deliverance from the end of another day of rounds.

Out in the hallway, Hannan was just about to walk into his secretary's office when he suddenly turned and headed back for A room where, he just remembered, he had seen something that needed his immediate attention. He pushed open the door and went directly to baby Fisher's warming table. On a stand, next to the table, sat Hannan's latest technological acquisition, a transcutaneous PO_2 monitor, a device that could monitor an infant's blood oxygen level by simply attaching a sensing device to the surface of the baby's skin. With the $TCPO_2$ monitor it would be possible to follow oxygen levels constantly, without having to draw a blood sample for analysis in the lab. The use of such a device, it was hoped, might someday help eliminate retrolental fibroplasia (RLF), a condition that used to lead to blindness in hundreds of tiny prematures because the high concentrations of oxygen needed to keep them alive also damaged the still-developing blood vessels in their eyes. The incidence of RLF has been greatly reduced by the careful monitoring and control of blood oxygen levels—something that was not possible in the past—but there is now some evidence that it can never be completely eliminated because some infants are simply more sensitive to oxygen than others. A device such as the $TCPO_2$ monitor, however, makes it possible to so closely follow, and therefore reduce or increase, oxygen levels that it may be possible to further reduce the number of RLF cases.

What Hannan was looking for and knew he wouldn't find was something to indicate that the nurses were regularly recording the data produced by the new monitor. "Where's this kid's data? I wanted to check it. . . . By the way, what's your name?" asked Hannan, who had not yet been formally introduced to Susie Phillips.

"Susie."

"Yell at me first, she's new," said Mabel Parrington, who was standing behind Hannan. Mabel was the unit's nurse-coordinator, the person responsible for the nursing program and staff in the unit.

"Yell at you? Okay. How are we recording the data for the transcutaneous PO_2s?"

"We're not."

"There ought to be some way of recording it."

"You mean on the sheet?" asked Mabel.

"Ya. How do I know the transcutaneous PO_2 and arterial PO_2 if it isn't being recorded?

"I have no idea, Jim, until we set up a system for it."

"We've got a system set up for recording it later on," Hannan told her.

"I haven't been in on any discussions of what we're going to do," said Mabel. "We can have a seperate sheet for it."

"Well, I think while the thing's being used, we ought to have some idea of what we're getting," Hannan told her. "While we were trying out the other oxygen monitors, we were writing down the data on the blood gas sheets."

"I have a system for that, and it will be written on the blood gas sheet and it will be written every fifteen minutes," said Hannan.

"It's still a new thing," said Mabel, "and no one knows what they're doing with it."

"We have to write it some place where I can find it and get it. Maybe we should just ask the nurse to write it in. I'll tell you what, I'd like it recorded just prior to any blood gas"—this was in order to compare the results of the measurement through the skin and the actual blood analysis in the lab—"and every time the alarm goes off."

"Who are you going to have sit there and write it down?"

"The nurse taking care of the baby."

"Not necessarily," warned Mabel."

"She can do that every fifteen minutes," Hannan told her.

"But she's not going to be doing it every fifteen minutes. She can watch it, but she's not going to be writing it down," said the nurse-coordinator, seeing her nurses about to have yet another responsibility dumped in their already overflowing laps.

"That's what I'm asking for. Just write it down," said Hannan, who wasn't prepared to give in on this issue.

"You can get respiratory therapy to come down and do it, but . . ." Mabel began.

"I'm asking that that recording be made, Mabel. Every fifteen minutes."

"And I'm asking that respiratory therapy come down and do it," she countered.

"You want respiratory therapy to come down every fifteen minutes?" Hannan asked, incredulous.

"If you've got a baby that's got to have it every fifteen minutes then you've got to have somebody other than the nurse. If it's *that* important, then we're probably talking about a baby who's very unstable."

"What's the sense of having the monitor, then, if the data isn't going to be recorded?" Hannan asked, a hard edge creeping into his tone.

"I said when you bought the thing that we didn't have the nurses."

"Look. It's only for two to four hours at a time. The thing shouldn't be on continuously. I think if a baby like this one has got one-to-one, or one-to-one-point-five nursing, you . . ."

"This baby's got one-to-two," Mabel corrected him.

"Then one-to-two. There should certainly be somebody looking at the baby at least every fifteen minutes, 'cause that baby's on a monitor and sick and so forth."

"This has got to be a team," said Mabel. "You can't dump it all on the nurses." Her voice remained even, but she was obviously agitated.

"It's not dumped on the nurses; it's part of nursing observation," Hannan told her.

"It's part of respiratory therapy," countered Mabel. The discussion was begining to sound a bit like a child's "Will not! Will so!" debate.

"Look, let's get respiratory therapy and talk to them," said Hannan. "I don't want to get into a fight with you, but this is gonna get done, one way or the other."

"And I'm asking for respiratory therapy to assist."

"You can ask respiratory therapy, but you're going to have to set it up. You have to draw up the plans and arrange it. If you want them to come down to do it every half-hour, fine. Why don't you draw up a policy?"

"I'm not drawing up any policy, because we don't need it," Mabel told him. "I'm just telling you you're not going to dump it all on the nurses."

"I'm *not* dumping it all on the nurses. I'm just telling you what I want, and I don't care how you get it. I'm just saying I want the measurements every fifteen minutes while the kid's on the monitor. You draw up a policy, work it out with respiratory therapy however you like. But as far as I'm concerned, it's a nursing observation, just like the monitor, heart rate, and so on. It's the same thing."

"They don't check that every fifteen minutes."

"On a sick baby? How often then?"

"The nurse has got a lot to do. Maybe every hour."

"I want the alarm on. How come the alarm isn't on?" asked Hannan, suddenly noticing that the new monitor's alarm was turned off.

"We haven't even had the in-service training on the thing yet," Mabel told him.

"I'm talking about all this for after the in-service's been done," said Hannan. "I'll draw up the policy and then you figure out how you're going to implement it." He ended the argument by turning on his heel and walking out, slamming the nursery door behind him.

Mabel Parrington stood by the warming table, watching Hannan's back recede quickly down the hall. "The nurses'll do it! The nurses'll do it! Write an order in the book and the nurses will do it. The medical staff couldn't do this? Of course they couldn't. They couldn't learn to write down a number, to calibrate the thing . . ." Her fuming was cut short by Evie Roth, who had been working nearby and had overheard the entire set-to.

"It never changes," the younger nurse commiserated. "I was stabilizing a baby an hour ago and one of the Fellows had the nerve to come up to me and ask me for a different style of stethoscope. Jesus! Out the window, buddy!"

Chapter Four

"If anyone wants me, I'll be down in the conference room," Jim Hannan told his secretary. "I'll be on page." He reached behind his inner-office door and grabbed a white lab coat that he pulled on as he walked. Already ten minutes late for the weekly educational rounds, Hannan turned right beyond the door and headed toward the stairs, rather than toward the antique elevators. He looked forward to the Friday-morning sessions and the pure intellectual challenge they provided, although he knew some members of his staff considered them a drag. Hannan always found the give and take of the discussions an excellent opportunity to measure the knowledge of his Fellows, residents, and medical students and to gauge their ability to think on their feet, freed of the pressures of the nursery.

By the time Hannan reached the first-floor conference room, the session was already well under way. Grabbing one of the three remaining donuts from the tray by the coffee urn and filling a styrofoam cup with black coffee, he took a seat back from the conference table, along the side wall of the room. Dr. Roberto DeLuca, the hospital's former director of education, was in midsentence, discussing the disparity between improvements in maternal survival rates and improvement in neonatal survival rates in the United States during the twentieth century.

"And this probably is one of the reasons why in seventy years we've made significant progress in saving mothers but have not made the same progress in saving the fetus, particularly from intrauterine deaths: We really know nothing about the bloody thing. Only a few obstetricians are interested in having autopsies performed on stillborns, and furthermore. . ."

"Pathologists, forgive me for interrupting, are bored to tears by these cases," cut in John Watkins, one of the two other fully trained neonatologists on Hannan's staff.

"This makes me mad! This makes me so mad!" continued De-Luca, whose brilliance was sometimes masked by his still-heavy Italian accent. "Every time I am on a committee they think that the autopsy of such babies is meaningless. Not only meaningless, but usually performed two weeks after delivery, and performed in a sloppy way. And there's no information whatever." Hannan's hand went up. "Yes, Jim?"

"Although I tend to agree with your comments, I think it's fair on balance to point out that animal studies suggest that the causes associated with acute and subacute asphyxia *in utero* are extraordinarily variable, and that the kinds of information you'd like to have would not come from a classical pathologist, but from a very good histopathologist and histobiochemist. The classical techniques are useless. So although I resent the attitude of physicians who don't order autopsies, I can't say that I get terribly excited when an autopsy wasn't done using classical techniques. The only possible use I've found, and of course this isn't often done, is to have somebody look microscopically at the liver, the pancreas, and the bone marrow to see if you're dealing with diabetic gestation."

"I fully agree with you," said DeLuca, who only contributed

to the educational conferences because of his respect for Hannan. His university had severed its ties with Metropolitan when it became apparent that the maternity hospital wasn't about to remain just an extension of the university's obstetrics department. But DeLuca learned from Hannan, just as the younger Hannan learned from him, so DeLuca managed to keep academic politics divorced from his teaching and learning relationships at Metropolitan. "A gross anatomical description is practically of little significance," DeLuca continued. "As you said, we must get a biochemical and analytical method for the pathological case. This is going to be very difficult, but we must look for drugs and chemicals that are present in the stillbirth."

DeLuca then pulled down a screen and, after one of the two St. Francis medical students in attendance turned off the lights, showed a slide of the declining maternal death rate during this century in the United States. "In the begining of the century, one lady out of 1,000 used to die in a delivery. Today, in this country, we have twenty to thirty-five deaths per 100,000 deliveries, a significant drop. We still have difficulties, as you know. The rate for nonwhites is higher than the rate in the white population.

"But as you can see," he said, gesturing toward the screen with a wooden pointer, "there hasn't been the same drop in the fetal death rate, or in the infant mortality rate. One of the reasons is that it's difficult to take care of a patient, like the fetus, who is inside the uterus. Until fifteen years ago we didn't have any kind of methodology to get inside until we got amniocentesis." Amniocentesis is the technique of using a needle to tap through the mother's abdomen, into the uterus, to withdraw a small sample of the amniotic fluid surrounding the fetus. Through an analysis of fetal cells in the fluid, physicians can now detect some genetic conditions, including sickle-cell anemia, Down's Syndrome, and Tay-Sachs disease. An analysis of the fluid can also be a help in determining the fetus's state of maturity and the development of its lungs.

As was his wont, Hannan was unprepared to accept DeLuca's

blanket statement about improvements in maternal survival. "We all see that slide at every meeting we go to," he told the obstetrician, "and we just sit there. But has anybody done a regression analysis to see whether the slope is significantly different at different times? Obviously, going from one per thousand to point two per thousand, or whatever, is significant. But has anybody ever looked at it by decades? I've never seen that. I've never seen these curves subjected to statistical analysis in the traditional sense. I've always seen statements like, 'We've dropped by this percent or that percent.' It sort of reminds me of the way economists tell us how good we're doing—'Inflation only rose by such and such a percentage this year.' Well so what?"

"What statistical hypothesis would you advance?" asked DeLuca.

"I'd like to know, for instance, whether the decade is the common yardstick," said Hannan. "Is there a significant difference in mortality between decades? I'd like to know what the equation looks like, because I think everybody would agree that there are probably several cycles that have occurred. I know every year these statistics are published in *Pediatrics*, but I've never seen them subjected to analysis."

"That's a very good objection, and we can call Atlanta and ask Dick Kranz at the Center for Disease Control. He must have done it.

"But let's move along," said DeLuca, who could see the session starting to disintegrate into a mathematical debate. "How did obstetricians approach this problem of fetal death? They approached it from a medical point of view. As you know, there is enough clinical experience to know a pregnancy is at risk when there is a bad family obstetrical history. We know very well that those who have had a stillbirth in the family, or a patient who has had a previous stillbirth, has a tendency of stillbirth. We know that socioeconomic status is correlated, for numerous reasons to poor pregnancy outcome, to medical complications, and to specific obstetrical complications, like pregnancy-induced hypertension. We knew that. Practically every obstetrician knew that. But only recently have we tried to put the thing together, to find out how *much* that pregnancy is at risk.

"At a number of centers," DeLuca continued, "on the West Coast, in Cleveland, Vermont, and here in particular, we have tried to develop a prenatal risk code. We've been using this code in our clinic here at Metropolitan. It's simple, and it's very arbitrary. The risk factors are ranked and each is given a number. When the patient comes for prenatal care, she is checked for each factor and receives a number total that should draw attention to how risky the pregnancy is. What does it mean that there's a prenatal risk code? You can see there's a correlation between the high- and low-risk code and the perinatal mortality [death occurring before, during, or up to twenty-eight days after birth]. In addition to the prenatal risk code, we have evaluated the intrapartum risk code, and, as you can see, the two high-risk scores, prenatal and intrapartum, are associated with the highest perinatal mortality. What I want to tell you is that these kinds of risk factors are very rough, very arbitrary, but that they draw attention, give you an indication of how risky the pregnancy may be. What do we know about these socioeconomic factors? Not really anything! We just know the problem has many factors."

"We do know the leading indicator of poor outcome is socioeconomic factors, not medical factors," said Hannan.

Although there are several different types of scales, scores, and systems for determining which obstetrical patients are likely to deliver a dead fetus, or which patient will deliver one of the 232,000 low-birthweight babies (infants weighing less than 2,500 grams, or 5.5 pounds, at birth) born in this country each year, the answers to five questions are far more important in determining outcome than are the total scores obtained from any tests.

"The questions," DeLuca told the group, "are: Is the fetus malformed? Is the fetus growing normally? Is the fetus in distress? How much metabolic reserve does the fetus have? And is the fetus capable of extrauterine life? This slide is old, but it's the slide I use to teach. I say, 'Did you answer number one? Number two? Number three? Number four? Number five?' "

"Number six: Do you tell the mother?" quipped Hannan, and the room filled with laughter.

"This is a really tough set of questions," said DeLuca. "It's difficult! The fetus," or *feetoos*, as he pronounced it, "is there. It's inside. But you don't know what to do. Up until recently we couldn't do anything for it. Now we can do something, but not very much. As you know, congenital abnormalities [so-called birth defects], in a general population, are two percent depending upon how you define congenital abnormalities. Two babies out of one hundred will have some kind of congenital abnormality. You know, for you to remember, a good rule is the rule of fives. The chromosomal abnormalities in spontaneous abortion, stillbirth, and live birth are fifty percent, five percent, and point five percent respectively. So, what do we do? As you know, at the present time we can detect chromosomal abnormalities and a small number of metabolic conditions. But we don't really know how medically to handle these mothers. We have arbitrarily said that even if there is no family history of these problems, we will put a needle in the belly of the mother at thirty-five years of age because there is an increased risk of Down's, and up to ninety-six percent of chromosomal abnormalities are Down's Syndrome," commonly referred to as mongolism.

"At the present time in obstetrics, for mothers aged thirty-five or older, we recommend amniocentesis to detect chromosomal abnormalities, and at the same time we do an alpha feto protein, because we have the fluid." About 3.5 percent, or almost double the usual rate, of babies born to mothers over thirty-five have congenital malformations, Deluca reminded the group. "Besides chromosomal abnormalities, besides neuro tubal defects [openings in the spinal column such as spina bifida] our main problem remains congenital heart disease. What is the incidence of congenital heart disease in the population at large?"

"Forty-seven per thousand?" volunteered Watkins, somewhat hesitantly.

"I like that number," said DeLuca. "Forty-five, forty-seven, somewhere in there. That is our main concern at the moment, and we know very little about that. Alpha feto proteins. How good is that? It's pretty good. Pretty good, but not exceedingly good. The main problem encountered in practice is that the amniotic fluid may give you exceedingly high results because you may have punctured the baby. Remember, alpha feto protein is the main protein in the plasma of the fetus and probably serves the same function as albumin in early fetal stages. And if you remember that fetal plasma is on the order of milligrams, and that in the amniotic fluid it's in micrograms, if just a smidgen of plasma goes from the fetal circulation into the amniotic fluid, your alpha feto protein there will shoot up [indicating an opening in the spinal column]. Always remember, this relationship is in micrograms, something like ten to the minus three. This is an extremely important issue. If you want to do an alpha feto protein in the mother, and the same time you want to do amniocentesis, the sample of maternal plasma has to be collected first, and the amniocentesis done afterwards. Because if you do the amniocentesis first, there is a passage of amniotic fluid into the maternal circulation, and this gives you a much higher reading of alpha feto protein in the maternal blood. Until this was understood, it was a significant problem. Another problem is that much of the result is directly related to the quality of the lab work. There are a lot of borderline values nobody knows how to treat. The absolute value, therefore, is not that important. What you must look for is a number two-and-one-half times the clinical value.

"Additionally," he continued, "it has been our experience that fifty percent of the samples you get are maternal contamination.

As far as I'm concerned, I can pick up only major changes in fetal growth. I can pick up significant, important, changes for the well-being of the fetus."

"The problem lies with clinic medicine," interrupted Hannan, "where you have different people seeing the patient each week, so there's no continuity. And you have people coming out of residency programs thinking the size of the uterus is not that important, when it's really one of the most important indicators."

"If I see the patient throughout pregnancy, I have two main indications of fetal growth," said DeLuca. "The first is the absolute value of the uterus. Twenty-eight centimeters is about twenty-eight weeks. This is less reliable than the slope of growth. It is less reliable than if I see a patient today and she is twenty-eight centimeters, and then I see her in four weeks and she is still twenty-eight. Then, independent of the number, I know the fetus is not growing."

"There is one use for that uterine length," said Hannan, as two St. Francis medical students and a first-year resident busily took notes, "and that is in the dialogue between obstetrician and neonatologist about whether a delivery should be done, or should you try to hold it off. Frequently one of my last questions to the obstetrician is, 'How big do you think the baby is?' And that becomes the moment of truth. He'll say, 'Well, he really feels a little small,' or 'Not a bad size.' And that's the only use I have for uterine length."

"The point is, I call that the estimated size of the baby," said Watkins, joining the dialogue. "Weight is something that really doesn't have any part in that discussion. All these other things fit very nicely. You really are doing something during an examination: You're feeling the baby's head somehow; you're feeling how long the baby is from head to toe."

"If you can hear the fetal heart with a normal stethoscope, you have to say the baby is at least twenty weeks at that point," said DeLuca.

"But you're doing something else, too," continued John Watkins. "You're touching the fetus within. You're not just saying, 'This is the height of the fundus'; you're saying, 'I can feel something within that uterus.' But it isn't weight you're feeling; it has something to do with length, head volume . . ."

"As you can see, from one patient to another the variability is just enormous," said DeLuca, picking up the thread of his lecture. "But if you look, there is a progression. And if you watch the progression, you have an indication of growth. I don't remember how many obstetricians, just before birth, during labor and delivery, look at the mother's belly and guess the fetal weight. And then they see the actual weight of the baby at delivery. As you can see," he said, gesturing with his pointer toward a slide, "when the baby weighs six point six pounds, the range of guesses is high and low, but they're all within a pound. When the baby is very big—ten point one—everybody tends to guess a little less. And, most important—*most important*—is a significant problem we are having when the baby is small, three point five pounds. Everybody tends to think that the unborn baby is a little bit bigger than it actually is. The result is that they urge delivery too early or fail to properly prepare for such a birth." Here he tapped the projection screen for emphasis.

"I know the objection of my friend, Jim," he continued, to a burst of laughter from those in the room. "Here is a dichotomy: We know very well that gestational age and probability of survival are, at the present time, different in the minds of different obstetricians, because obstetrics today is a branch of medicine in development. The fetus is at a cutoff point. It was not uncommon ten years ago to see an obstetrician write off a baby of thirty-one, thirty weeks. And it is not uncommon today, even in this hospital among senior staff, to write off a baby who is twenty-nine, twenty-eight weeks. I don't think there are many in this hospital who consider the fetus an entity at twenty-six weeks. Am I correct?"

"Not many," said Hannan, bitterly.

"So we must consider there is a progression in fetal development," said DeLuca.

"But there's a logical inconsistency there," said Hannan. "The neonatal service is only going to be as good as the obstetrical service. Projected inability to survive becomes a self-fulfilling prophecy. And that's what happens to the lower end of the survival curve."

"I know," agreed DeLuca, "it's a dichotomy. But let's move on. How good is sonogram?" he asked, referring to the use of sound waves, or ultrasound, to create a picture of the fetus while still in the uterus.

"When? Where?" asked Hannan, typically refusing to accept even the most basic question or statement at face value.

"How good is the sonogram, and when and where should it be used?" DeLuca rephrased his question.

"Good enough to place you within three days of gestational age," said Watkins.

"The sonogram has been a significant improvement in obstetrical management, there is no doubt," said DeLuca. "The management of placenta previa? God! I can't think of the times we used to have a double setup to examine and make diagnosis of placenta previa," he said, referring to a condition in which the placenta lies across the opening of the cervix and can therefore begin bleeding, possibly proving fatal to both mother and fetus. "We'd have everybody ready to do a cesarean section and have the lady in the delivery room. It was a nightmare, with everybody ready with the knife. If a lady now comes in, and she bleeds a little bit, nobody touches her and you send her down for a sonogram. If the sonogram shows no central placenta previa, or partial placenta previa, God, it's an improvement, if you think that at one time placenta previa was diagnosed by internal examination. And when the bleeding started in the old time, you know what we used to do? Reach for the baby's legs, do an internal rotation through the placenta, bring the baby's feet down, and pull it out! Sacrifice the baby to save the mother. I can give you a book written in 1914, in which it is mentioned that a good obstetrician should have a salvage rate of the mother, using this maneuver for placenta previa, of about six percent." The room was filled with gasps and cries of "God!" "The progress has been significant in this respect, and sonograms have made a big contribution to this.

"Now, to estimate fetal growth, we follow it by measuring biparietal diameter [the size of the skull]."

"The thing that's always bothered me," said Hannan, "and yet obstetricians have never bothered to tackle it, is that the preponderance of the animal experimentation and human clinical data suggests that nature, in its wisdom, preserves head growth at the expense of everything else. So, the point I'm trying to make is that by the time you see reduced head size, the ball game is pretty much lost. That or you're dealing with a different population of intrauterine growth retardation from what we see outside the uterus. Because what we usually see when we get them are scrawny kids with normal-size heads."

"Gestational age is essential to understand for two main reasons," DeLuca explained, taking over again. "One is to evaluate fetal growth, particularly in the third trimester. The second is to establish the time of post date. These are our two main issues. The criteria that you use are the last menstrual period and the physical examination at first visit. If you go in a certain tiny examination room here and you examine a patient for the size of the uterus, and you turn your head ninety degrees, you will find on the wall . . ." DeLuca paused for an instant, waiting for Hannan to stop chuckling at what the neonatologist knew was coming ". . . that I wrote the size of the uterus at different gestational ages. I made that for the students, so they could tell, by comparing the size, what week of pregnancy the woman was in. And you will remember, for your information, that at eight weeks the uterus is a pear, at ten weeks it is an orange, at twelve weeks a grapefruit, at fourteen weeks a coconut, and, if you want, at sixteen weeks a pineapple."

"In size only," said Hannan.

"And in shape," DeLuca corrected him. "This is what I am trying to tell you. In the first trimester you can make a mistake of one week only. In the second you do a sonogram. When do you do it? The first sonogram should be at sixteen, seventeen, eighteen weeks. If she comes in early, it's very easy to estimate. If she comes in at twenty weeks, it's very difficult. If there is no prenatal care, you don't know where you are.

"Well, that about takes up our hour. We have a few more items to discuss: How to tell fetal distress, how much reserve the fetus has, and lung maturation."

"We'll get you back again," said Hannan, rising from his chair.

"I'd be delighted," said DeLuca. "I think this kind of two-way discussion is the best way to exchange information."

"Jesus!" thought Hannan. "If only we could exchange this much information with half our obstetricians." As he headed back up for the nursery, Hannan began thinking over what De-Luca had said about the progress made in this century in the quality of obstetric care. One's definition of progress, he often thought, depends on what one is trying to improve. Too often the obstetricians viewed the health and safety of the mother as the only thing they needed to consider. Oh, he realized that wasn't entirely fair, but they sure as hell didn't give as much thought to the baby as to the mother. How many times had he found out about some OB who had taken some lady at less than thirty weeks and, because the baby would be born dead or die right away anyway, had given drugs to induce labor, put the mother to sleep, and used forceps to "empty the uterus," never bothering to call the Code Pink team. And the thirty-weeker would invariably turn out to be thirty-three weeks and then someone would put in a hurried call to the nursery, but the baby would be a wreck by the time help arrived. He wasn't kidding when he'd told Roberto that the neonatal service could be only as good as the obstetric service. If the OBs would let the Code Pink team know when they had a mother in early labor, then something could be done. If they'd consult, for God's sake! There was no question things were improving. Hell, in 1970, 14 percent of the babies born at Metropolitan and weighing between 500 and 1,000 grams (1.1 and 2.2 pounds) survived. In 1976, 41 percent of the babies born in that weight category at Metropolitan survived. If you looked at the current 750-to-1,000-gram group, the nursery's rate jumped to almost ninety percent, well above the national average.

The quality of care of premature infants has come an incredibly long way since Chicago's Michael Reese Hospital opened the nation's first premature infant center in 1922. Today, throughout the United States, there are more than 500 such centers, saving babies who only a decade ago were, in all but a handful of centers, thought of as miscarried fetuses, rather than premature infants with a chance of living—and of living a normal life.

How many babies are born at risk each year? How likely is the average mother to bear a baby either weighing less than 5½ pounds, or suffering from a life-threatening condition before its life even begins? How relevant, in other words, is the work of Jim Hannan and his team at Metropolitan Lying-In to most mothers-to-be? Far too relevant.

Although estimates differ, it is generally believed that about one in every seven of the 3.3 million infants born in the United States each year is born at risk. The figure varies from city to city and from region to region. A 1978 study by the Robert Wood Johnson Foundation found, for instance, that an estimated 27.5 percent of the infants born in the entire state of Arizona can be considered at high risk, while only 10 percent of the babies born in Cleveland, Ohio, and its four contiguous counties fall into that category. While thousands of middle-class women suffer through the experience of having a baby's life hang in the balance in an intensive care nursery, there is no question that, as Roberto De-Luca and Jim Hannan pointed out, poverty clearly plays a part in producing high-risk infants. That same Robert Wood Johnson study found wide variations in the percentage of high-risk infants born in three regions of Los Angeles, and those percentages range from 22 percent in part of Los Angeles that is 22 percent nonwhite to 33 percent in an area 36 percent nonwhite to an astounding 73 percent in an area 60 percent nonwhite. And the variation has nothing to do with race per se, experts believe, but rather is correlated in some way to the numerous variables associated with poverty—variables including lack of proper prenatal care, women under age seventeen giving birth, more smoking and drinking, drug use, poor housing conditions, lack of proper diet, hypertension, diabetes, anemia, and, perhaps, the very stress that is so much a part of urban life for all and is particularly magnified for the poor. While many of these same factors contribute to prematurity in middle-class women, poor women are far more likely to have many of these problems simultaneously.

Living in or near a sophisticated urban area is no guarantee that an infant born at risk will receive proper care. Washington D.C., the nation's capital, has had, for at least the past decade, either the worst—or the second- or third-worst—urban infant mortality rate in the country. This situation wasn't even considered a major public health problem until late 1978, two years after *The Washington Post* began carrying articles and editorials about it. As is often the case in other areas, Washington's public health officials, who recognized that there was a problem, consistently blamed it on the city's high teenage pregnancy rate and on the fact that many of the city's poor women were getting little or no prenatal care. Even in the face of a detailed study of infant deaths in 1977, a study that showed that teenage pregnancy had very little to do with the staggeringly high infant mortality rate, these officials continued to argue that city programs designed to reduce infant mortality should focus on reducing teenage pregnancy.

However, a recent study by the National Capital Medical Foundation, the city's federally chartered physician peer-review group, finally laid some of the myths to rest. At the same time it may have shattered the complacency of many middle-class women who believed that they were immune from perinatal problems for they, after all, went to respected private hospitals. That study found that over 90 percent of the newborn infants who died in Washington in 1977 weighed less than 2,500 grams at birth. They were, by definition, born at risk. But what was particularly horrifying was the wide variation in mortality rates at different hospitals: The best hospital in the city saved 54 percent of the babies born weighing between 500 and 1,000 grams, while the next-best, a private university teaching hospital, saved only about 33 percent. Another university hospital had less than a 25 percent survival rate for infants in the same weight group, and D.C. General Hospital, the city's municipal hospital, had about an 86 percent *mortality* rate—it saved only *14 percent* of the babies in the same weight category in which the best hospital saved 54 percent.

The study, which examined the care the dead infants received in the hospital, painted a picture that can only suggest that these very low birthweight babies are being written off as unsavable in hospitals just a few miles from the National Institutes of Health, and only blocks from the seat of the federal health establishment. Among the study's more shocking findings:

• An astounding 14 percent of the babies who died were born in a hospital but outside a delivery room. They were born as their mothers lay in ward beds, labor rooms, hallways, or waiting rooms.

• About 40 percent of the mothers given general anesthesia were not intubated; that is, they did not have a tube placed in their trachea to ensure that the oxygen they were being given actually reached their lungs, and thus their babies. Failing to intubate such a patient, say some nationally know experts in obstetrical anesthesia, consitutes medical malpractice in and of itself.

Those conducting the study conducted a special, even more detailed, examination of the care given 106 infants who died but who—because they weighed more than 500 grams, breathed for at least one hour, and had no lethal malformations—might have had a reasonable chance to survive. They found that:

• Over 53 percent of those infants had not been tested for the pH (acidity) of their blood, a prerequisite to deciding on the kind of chemical and drug aids the infant might need.

• Forty percent of the babies born with low Apgar scores, a scoring system designed to evaluate the baby's respiratory, pulmonary, and neurological functioning, were not given any oxygen in the delivery room, a lapse akin to seeing a baby bleeding to death at an accident scene and not helping.

• Almost 20 percent of the infants who were cyanotic (blue from a lack of oxygen and excess of carbon dioxide in the blood) were not given oxygen in the nursery.

• Over 63 percent of the infants did not have their blood sugar levels tested, a necessity for deciding on a proper course of treatment.

• Over 53 percent of the infants never had their blood pressure taken.

From looking at the numbers, one gets the clear impression that those 106 babies died, or at least were never given a reasonable chance of living, because they were not expected to live. If you expect a baby to live, if you want it to live, you give it oxygen if it is turning blue. If its heart is not beating, or it is having difficulty breathing, you resuscitate it. This does not suggest that the physicians involved wanted the babies to die. Rather they, and thousands of physicians around the nation, were trained in a day when such babies didn't live no matter what was done for them. Such deaths were unavoidable. And in many American hospitals they are still unavoidable, for neonatal intensive care units often have to compete for dollars and staff (which is another way of saying dollars) with other, better-known, more visible intensive care units, like those for heart attack victims. And parents who have had, now have, or will have babies in intensive care nurseries, are, as Jim Hannan tells all his Fellows and students, episodic users of the health-care system. Once their baby either lives or dies, they no longer have contact with the hospital. They feel no need to pressure hospital boards or elected officials to improve facilities. On the other hand, the relative of a heart attack victim knows full well that he himself may one day need a bed in a cardiac care unit. He wants to be sure that there will be enough such beds when the time comes.

And thus, as he stood waiting for one of the elevators that never seemed to come at Metropolitan Lying-In, Jim Hannan continued to think about Roberto DeLuca's comment about progress. "Maybe I really should chuck it all and go be a fishing guide in Montgomery County," he thought, shaking his head as he finally stepped into the elevator.

Chapter Five

"Look at that, will you," Mary Anne whispered to Susie. "He hasn't moved for the last hour. He just sits there rocking, staring at the baby. They practically ran him over during rounds, but he didn't budge."

"I think it's sweet," the younger nurse said, a little too loud for the close quarters in the nursery.

"Well, I think it's weird," Mary Anne shot back. "I mean, it's terrific that he seems to care so much about the baby, but he gives me the creeps, just sitting there like that. You'd think he was keeping an eye on us to make sure we don't hurt the kid."

"Maybe he is."

"I just wish he'd go do his job and let us do ours. He's really getting under my skin," Mary Anne replied angrily, making a notation on her clipboard and turning away from Susie in the same motion.

Robert Durand had been oblivious to the nurses' conversation, as he always was to what went on in the nursery around him. He had taken brief notice of the crowd surrounding him during rounds but had quickly tuned out Jim Hannan's recital of the baby's condition. He had heard the details so many times he could have given the presentation himself.

An executive with an international banking firm, Durand had always been a quiet man, speaking only when the need arose and then saying as little as possible. But this whole business with little Stephen had driven him even further into himself. He would ask questions of the doctors and nurses about his son's condition and then stare at them as they replied, his brown eyes unmoving, his fixed, enigmatic smile giving no hint of how he was reacting to their information. He would then thank them politely and return to his rocking, changing position either to place his hands on his tiny son as the baby slept in his Isolette, or to draw them back out through the twin portholes. "You will be fine," he thought to himself in his native French. "You see. Soon we will take you home from this place where they are always poking you and sticking you with needles. We will be together, as a family should be. You are a strong little boy. Before you know it it will be summer and we will all fly to Nice to visit your grandparents. You will be big and strong by then. We will all walk together on the beach and . . ."

"Robert?" A hand lightly touched his shoulder from behind and he looked up to see his wife, Jessica, standing beside him. She moved her hand from his shoulder to his forehead as he looked up, stroking a stray lock of black hair out of his eyes.

"How is he doing?" she asked, looking down at the baby—her son—who seemed, as he lay in his plexiglass cage, more the property of the hospital than her own flesh and blood. She still half-expected to come in one morning and find a metal label attached to the bottom of one of his feet, like the ones she saw on all the equipment: "Property of Metropolitan Hospital. Do Not Remove. 0901478."

"He's doing better today," Robert told her. "Jim said he had a good night. They may begin to taper off some of the medication if things stay this smooth."

Durand rose from the white nursery rocking chair and prepared to return to work, as his wife busied herself with the toys and gadgets with which the couple had surrounded their infant son. She saw that the tape recorder had shut itself off and rewound the tape, Pachelbel's *Canon in D*. That done, she started the recorder again, filling the baby's Isolette—via a tiny pillow speaker—with the blissfully peaceful strains of the 300-year-old music. She had a hunch the night-shift nurses were using the recorder for something else, but she had no proof. If she ever got it, she thought, there was going to be some real hell to pay. If she couldn't have her baby, the least she could do was try to make him comfortable, to take him out of the hospital with music, if by no other way.

As soon as Robert had gathered up his things and left, promising to be home from work early so they could come back to the hospital together in the evening, Jessica Durand settled herself into the rocker warmed by her husband's body and, like him, began to stare. Her thoughts drifted back to the day five weeks ago when the nightmare that was their present life had begun. She was entering her twenty-seventh week of pregnancy; in fact, she had been to see her obstetrician, Joan Clark, just two days before, and everything had been normal.

Joan had asked when she and Robert were going to start childbirth classes, and Jessica had explained that they were not to start for another two weeks. Robert was even more excited than she about the prospect of his being in the labor and delivery rooms, Jessica had told Joan. The classes would be fun, and they would also make this whole business of pregnancy seem a bit more real. It was hard to realize she was going to have a baby when she hadn't even experienced any morning sickness, or a craving for so much as a single pickle.

But two mornings later she had awoken with a slight discharge. Nothing to be alarmed about, she thought, just a dampness where there should be none. She had forgotten the incident by lunchtime and hadn't even mentioned it to Robert. At a party that evening, however, as she stood sipping a glass of club soda, she sensed that something was amiss. She had gone into the ladies' room and discovered that the discharge had grown quite heavy. But still, she wasn't alarmed. Two friends of hers who happened to be in the ladies' room at the same time, older women who had together experienced seven pregnancies and six births, weren't alarmed either. "It's probably just the baby switching position and squeezing on your bladder," one of them had told her. And she had believed because she had wanted to.

She didn't have any discharge the following day and had even walked the fifteen blocks to her office in the bright, crisp fall morning. She was exhausted by noon but attributed that to her walk. "A nap is all I need," she thought, taking advantage of the couch in the office ladies' room. She was still tired when she awoke an hour later, and by the end of the day she could barely move. But she had promised to meet Robert at a downtown department store to shop for baby furniture. "We have to get that room ready," she had thought. "I'll go ahead and meet him and then let him fix me dinner for a change."

She had arrived at their meeting place about forty minutes early, and to this day, seven weeks later, she still could not remember much about the next forty minutes. "I know I went to the ladies' room," she had told a friend, "and the next thing I remember was leaning against the wall of the ladies' room, not with the waters breaking, but with a definite discharge. I was feeling totally out of touch with what was going on. Totally alone. There were thousands of people in the store, but not a soul there with me."

Somehow she had found her way back to the bank of elevators where she was supposed to meet Robert, and the next thing she remembered was throwing herself into his arms when he arrived at 7 P.M., crying, sobbing, "I can't do it! I just can't do it!"

"It's okay, it's okay!" Robert told her repeatedly. "We don't need to shop tonight. Let's go home."

The brief cab ride back to their rented townhouse was one she would never forget. She was experiencing excruciating back pains before the ride was half-over, and not knowing anything about labor or labor pains, she threw herself down on the floor when she got home and began doing the exercises she had found in a self-help pregnancy book, exercises intended for use during and after pregnancy. She thought the exercise would help ease the pain. Instead, she quickly felt as though somebody were kicking her with football cleats. By 9 P.M., when she could stand no more of the pain, with or without exercise, she gave up and called Joan Clark.

As she sat, rocking beside her son's Isolette in the ICN, she could still remember that conversation word for word. "Joan!" she had gasped. "There's something wrong. I—" she was stopped from completeing the sentence by another sharp pain.

"Don't try to say anything," Joan told her. "You're in labor. Just get to Metropolitan and I'll meet you there. You're in labor," she repeated.

Jessica could not believe her doctor's words. How could she be in labor? She was only twenty-seven weeks pregnant. She hadn't had any strenuous exercise, and she'd heard of women who even skied while they were pregnant! "There must be some mistake," she thought. But there was no mistaking the pain she felt, and within minutes she and Robert were back in a taxi, this time headed for Metropolitan Hospital. "What a nightmare," she recalled. "We just didn't know a thing. And at nine at night this hospital was like the set of a movie—*Hospital.* Those old gentlemen in the admitting office are nice enough, like somebody's old uncle. But they just don't know what labor pains are." She giggled quietly to herself as she continued rocking. "Maybe if they went through labor they wouldn't be so slow in registering you," she thought.

Joan Clark arrived at Metropolitan only moments after the Durands and was back to see Jessica in the labor room shortly after Jessica had been helped into a hospital gown and Clark had slipped on hospital greens. "We have to get a urine sample; can you give it to us? We have to know if there's amniotic fluid," her patient remembered being told. Jessica also remembered that, being doubled over in pain, she had replied, "You've got to be kidding!"

"Okay," Clark had told her, "we'll just put a catheter in."

"Oh no, you won't! You just help me down to the bathroom. I'll cooperate! I promise!"

"I thought you would," the doctor told her, and both women began laughing loudly, the tension dissolved for the moment.

Five weeks later, as Jessica sat watching her tiny son, lying on his back in the plexiglass Isolette , his skin a translucent pink, she felt a twinge of guilt over the fact that she had not thought about her baby during her labor. "How could I have forgotten you so?" she mused. "I didn't think beyond the pain. I didn't think about you until I saw you hours later. I came out of the bathroom and gave them that urine sample and they told me, you're going to give birth, and I still didn't believe it. I was fully dilated and I still didn't believe it. I knew your heart was fine, because they were monitoring you, but I didn't believe you were about to be born. Do you know what I said to a nice nurse who came over and asked if I had had childbirth classes yet? I said, 'No, I'm not that pregnant.' "

The nurse stayed with Jessica for the next hour, teaching her how to breath, helping her to ride the top of the waves of pain, what the Lamaze instructors call "discomfort." By the time Joan Clark announced at midnight that the birth was imminent, Jessica had things reasonably well under control. But she still refused, or was unable, to believe she was about to give birth. Even the delivery seemed unreal, she recalled. A whiff of oxygen, five minutes of pushing, and 1,180 grams of baby slipped from her vagina before she realized she was giving birth. And as fast as the baby appeared, he disappeared, swept up by the waiting Code Pink team.

While the work of the team is a wonder for the interested observer to behold, it can be bewildering, if not terrifying, for the mother lying on the delivery table. As Jessica thought about it later, she realized that although she felt removed from what was going on, she somehow expected to be handed a bouncing baby and to be surrounded by beaming nurses and doctors. But it didn't happen that way. Instead, the baby was taken by the team members working to save its fragile life. All Jessica could remember, as she thought back, was Javed holding the baby near her face for what seemed like half a second, asking, "Do you want to see the baby?" and then whisking him away as she turned to look. There wasn't, she would realize later, any time for amenities. "You didn't have any lungs," she thought as she watched Stephen, who was still sleeping. "You took one breath and then what will be your lungs collapsed. They just weren't ready yet. I didn't realize it then, but Javed saved your life. There's no question about that. He saved your life."

While Jessica was moving through the system, being cleaned up in the recovery room and readied for the trip to her third-floor room, her husband had gone to the ICN to see his first son. "Your daddy came into my room around one-thirty in the morning," she continued, thinking to the baby, "and right away, I knew something was wrong. Dr. Clark was with him, and the head nurse, and a nurse from the nursery. Joan said she was going to give me something to go to sleep, but I told them, 'No, you're not! I want to know what's going on.' Well, I don't know how Joan did it. But she handled it with so much grace, so much aplomb. By then it was almost three A.M., and she was obviously dead tired, but she also obviously wasn't going home until I understood what was happening. She told me what she felt and thought, and what Javed had told her. And then she said, 'Okay, if you want to go and see him, we won't try to stop you.' She was just totally on my side. Maybe she sensed how confused and scared your mommy was."

Jessica decided to sleep for a few hours before going up, convinced that if they were willing to let her see her baby, things couldn't possibly be as bad as she had originally imagined.

By the time she made her way upstairs about five hours later, the day-side nurses were already at work, and Jim Hannan was making his first pass-through of the day. "It was all so confusing," she recalled. "I remember coming through the scrub area, and the lights and the noise. I remember not really knowing where I was. I must have had tunnel vision, thinking, 'Okay, steer me where you want me to go, I don't want to look at anything else.' And, my God, when I finally got there and went to sit down, I'll never forget how that stool shot out from under me, and everyone rushed over like I'd fainted!

"And to see you lying there!" she thought, as though speaking to her sleeping infant. " I'd never seen anything so small, or felt such a wrenching in my stomach. I didn't think I could ever feel so many conflicting emotions as I did then. I just wanted to gather you up in my arms and take you out of there! You were surrounded by all this machinery, with these huge hands and tubes all over you. Your chest was the only thing moving, and that seemed so artificial. You looked like a horse with a bit with that Logan bar. You were just overwhelmed by all that paraphernalia, and I felt preempted. Maybe that's the wrong word, but I was definitely put on the sidelines. There was nothing I could do for you!" Her face clouded over as she again recalled how useless she felt beside the nurses—an outsider who did not really belong in their world.

"My God! I actually thought it would be better for him to die than lie there like that," she remembered painfully. "I had no idea what they had done to him. I didn't know what any of their jargon meant. I had no idea what his condition was. I just knew that this was my child and he was being kept alive, and what else? Jim came over to me and said he'd rather come down to the room and talk to me later. He told me I could touch you," she thought, resuming her imaginary conversation with Stephen, "and he said we could talk later. Do you know that for the next three or four days, every time I'd come in to see you I'd sit down on a stool, bury my head in my gown, and just cry? One of the nurses would always hand me a tissue on the sly, because they knew I'd be embarrassed if people knew I was crying. But there was nothing else I could do. The tears were uncontrollable."

Jessica's first reaction to Hannan was quite mixed. She thought him very matter-of-fact, kind, and gentle. But she was resentful of the very calmness for which she was grateful. "I hated it," she recalled as she rocked, now knitting a tiny blue sweater she had not started prior to Stephen's birth. "I thought, 'Why me? Why is this happening to us and why is this man taking it so calmly?' Jim is a pro, a crackerjack. He knows what he's doing. But, God! I resented him. I resented all the care the nurses were giving and I resented being literally put on the sidelines. I still do, for that matter! I felt totally out of touch with you," she thought, switching back to her one-way silent dialogue with Stephen. "You were accessible then, because you were on a table and not stuck in an Isolette. Because your condition was so bad you were out where they could get at you, so I could touch you, too."

Hannan had visited Jessica in her room about a half-hour after her brief initial visit to the nursery. He had explained hyaline membrane disease and the immediate threat it posed to Stephen. He explained that Stephen's patent ductus—the opening between the aorta and pulmonary artery that, in the fetus, is a main conduit of circulation but is meant to close at birth—hadn't closed as it should have, and he had some fluid buildup around his heart. As was his style, Hannan didn't pull any punches. He laid out all the problems facing the baby and the ways he thought he might be treated. "He did try to explain," recalled Jessica, "but the jargon, the language, is totally impossible to understand without some medical training. He tried to explain it as simply as he could, but it's just impossible. You simply can't understand all the ramifications of the problems. It took me several weeks to understand that Stephen basically had no lungs. I remember thinking, 'Well, they'll keep the tubes in for a couple of weeks and the machine will do its work and then he'll start breathing on his own.' But I just didn't understand. He didn't have lungs to start breathing with. The sacks were just flat. The tissue wasn't there. But Jim kept trying to explain. Every day I was in the hospital he'd come down several times and go over and over and over the same things until I understood them."

The Durands had felt it was their constant presence in the nursery that was annoying the staff, and, in part, they were right. But what had also rubbed raw many sets of nerves was the couple's overintellectualizing of their situation, a not-uncommon defense mechanism used by well-educated parents confronting such emotionally charged circumstances. Frequently, before visiting Stephen, Jessica would bury herself in the neonatology textbooks she found in the nursing lounge. She would devour every word about every symptom and change in Stephen's condition. She would question treatments and ask whether certain alternative treatments were being considered. If they weren't, she would want to know why. While the staff was pleased by the Durands' attempt to understand their son's illness and better cope with the reality of it, they were also irked by what some came to view as second-guessing by barely informed laymen, particularly in a field where the textbooks, and even some of the journals Jessica was reading, were months, if not years, behind the kind of fringe medicine being practiced in Metropolitan's ICN. And, as Jessica was thinking this Christmas Eve afternoon, while there were other parents who visited their babies frequently, she and Robert were coming close to setting a record for almost constant presence in the nursery. This was a record that didn't sit well with the nurses, no matter how much they said they appreciated parental involvement.

"Here I am, sitting here several times a day," she thought, watching a nurse draw blood from a baby in the next Isolette, "and there are babies who have been here three months whose parents I never see. I just don't think the staff will ever get used to my being here, and they're sure not going to get used to having a mother who's saying, 'Okay, I'll change him, he's my child. If he's not hooked up to a monitor, and I won't disturb anything, why can't I change him?' Working here takes a certain kind of personality. A lot of these nurses have children of their own, and they certainly have strong mothering instincts. I know not all of us have it, but most of these women certainly do. They see themselves as caretakers, and some of these babies who lie in the Isolettes and never see their parents, see only these women. The babies have three different mothers, one for each shift. I just don't understand these mothers who never come in. Some don't even call. But then I've never been sixteen or seventeen, single, and the mother of a two-pound baby. Look at little Louanne's mother. She must be about nineteen, no husband, another child. She obviously loves this baby; she just doesn't get in much. But then, I guess at her age she has other fish to fry. I can remember being nineteen, and a baby wasn't what I was thinking about, especially one I couldn't see most of the time. Coming in here just isn't at the top of her list of priorities. And I guess the number of visits is really no measure of love.

"But, my God," thought Jessica, "that baby is Susie's baby during the day, and Mildred's baby evenings, and Margaret's baby after eleven, and then it's somebody else's again in the morning. But I know that when they think of Stephen, they think of Robert and me—mention us in the same breath—so there has to be a conflict of some sort there. But the most important thing for us is to be here with Stephen now, while he needs us. Especially now that the steroids have really begun to do their work. His lungs are improving and it looks like he's going to make it. If I make a nuisance out of myself, so be it. If the staff isn't used to a mother and father who are both here several times a day, then so be it! But they were happy enough to have us during that blizzard two weeks ago. Our apartment is so close, and we've made the trip so many times, that I didn't even think about the fact that many of the nurses might not make it in. But the nursery was in a total panic when I got here. The night shift was still on and the day shift hadn't come in because of the snow. Robert managed to get over here when I called and told him about the staffing problem. And there we were, providing most of the care for the noncritical babies—feeding them, changing them, bathing them. I'll never forget Mary Anne's expression when she was getting ready to go eat, and she said, 'So-and-so, you watch this room, and so-and-so is sleeping down the hall, and Louise, you and I will go get something to eat. Oh! There's no one left to watch the other babies. Well, Mr. and Mrs. Durand are here. You can watch them, can't you?' And we said 'of course.' You know, Stephen," she said, switching her thoughts back to her son, "I've really come to love some of your little friends here. But I swear, it's like vying for title rights with some of these nurses. They just don't understand. No one can understand until they've had this happen to them. Even though these ladies taking care of you see this every day as their work, they've never thought about what it would be like if it happened to them. Like Betty. She always talks about having had a premature baby. But for God's sake! That was sixteen years ago. The child was one month premature and now she's a strapping young lady of five-feet-eight. Betty has no concept what this is like. If her daughter had been your size back then she would never have survived. There's just no understanding there. In fact, there's an implicit lack of understanding. Oh, they're involved with the critical, moment-to-moment drama of the situation," she paused, reaching into the Isolette to free Stephen's minute arm—an arm so frail she always feared breaking it—which had become entangled in a monitor lead, "but it's different when you're on the receiving end."

The thing that made these weeks incredibly hard, she often thought, was not so much Stephen's condition, as the uncertainty of that condition. She felt desolate, and the approach of Christmas, with its socially enforced joviality, did not make things any easier. She'd often find herself thinking, "It's Christmas time, my child is in the hospital, and I don't know if he's going to live. I just never expected any of this. I go to the hospital, I come home, and I realize that he's in a situation totally removed, totally alien to us. He's my own baby but he's living somewhere else. Why do I have to keep convincing myself that I've given birth? I do have a child! He's just not home with us now."

Through it all, Robert was a rock, never questioning, never doubting for a moment, that his son would survive to come home. He, like his wife, asked many questions of the doctors and nurses. But he always seemed more satisfied with the answers, readier to accept and digest the bit of knowledge imparted with each reply, less likely to follow every question with two more. As he and Jessica walked home from the hospital at night, he would be perfectly calm and she would be crying, tears literally streaming down her face.

"I just can't take another day of this!" she sobbed on more than one occasion. "Just let him be well or die!"

And Robert would stop walking, place his hands on her shoulders, look into her eyes, and say quietly, "Oh, no. He's going to be fine. You'll see. He will get bigger, and stronger, and one day soon we will take him home with us. You must not worry. It will be fine."

When this happened Jessica would find herself at once loving him for his strength and confidence, and hating what she saw as his smugness in the face of her insecurity. She wanted some of his strength but could not escape the image of Stephen the first morning she saw him, lying on the nursery table like some rag doll in the clutches of a mad scientist. Wires were attached to Stephen's nonexistent chest, which rose and fell to the pumping of the respirator. That image never left her. Never. She'd be happy for the little successes—the removal of one tube, or one wire, or the dropping of carbon dioxide levels and increase in his blood oxygen. But no matter how much better things got, that image would always remain.

The situation had done little to help Jessica and Robert's personal relationship. They were alternately withdrawing into themselves and leaning upon one another for support. Their sex life, she would laughingly tell a close friend, was nonexistent, a thing of the past. "One feels an intense guilt," she would say, "and that predisposes one to a lot of other emotions. Seeing the baby the way he is, feeling it's my fault—like, 'What have I done?'—makes it very hard to relax and focus on something else, like sex. We've put that out of our minds. Robert's never, *never* said anything to indicate that he blames me in any way. But there's nothing you can say to someone who's going to feel guilty to make them not feel guilty. I'm sure the guilt will dissipate after a while; it's lessening now, but it takes time."

For Stephen's first two weeks, when things looked particularly bleak as his lung disease developed, Jessica would find herself physically unable to get out of bed in the morning to face the trip to the hospital. She would lie in bed beside Robert, staring at the ceiling. "I just can't get out of this bed anymore," she would tell him. "Please do it for me. Please go to the nursery and come back and tell me everything's going to be all right. I can't put Stephen through this anymore! I know I'm being a coward." It all simply became too much to bear. She would see her son, blinders on his eyes to protect them from the ultraviolet light heating his jaundice, a respirator tube as large as his neck snaking across the table top, and she'd watch his condition fluctuate. One hour the respirator pressure was up, and the next it would be down. The oxygen was high and then the oxygen was low. And she would cringe as he was stuck, prodded, and moved around by the nurses with a seeming casualness Jessica could never understand. Had Stephen died that first week, she had thought it would be easy to accept, because he still wasn't real to her. He wasn't Robert's baby. He was, quite simply, the hospital's baby. Robert and Jessica tried to make Stephen theirs, doing what they could to establish their space around him. They surrounded him with toys, cluttering the area near the table. And when he was moved into the Isolette, they moved the toys in with him, making him look like a doll stuffed into a transparent toy chest. But they still didn't feel he was their baby.

As the days turned into weeks, and the weeks became the first month, Jessica also began to feel she was being cheated in some strange way she couldn't quite define. But she had always harbored certain fantasies about giving birth and about motherhood—fantasies destroyed by her going into labor almost twelve weeks early. As she sat watching Stephen in his toy-crammed Isolette she thought about those dreams lifted from the pages of women's magazines, dreams she would never realize, at least not with this pregnancy. "The mommy always gets to let her hair down," she thought. "She gets to relax. She brings the baby home and it's a piece of cake. But this . . . I'm always on call because he's so sick. I never know when a given moment will be his last. I can never relax. I've never had that period when I can say, 'Oh, I want to take a rest from this for a bit. My mind and body aren't ready for this. My hormones are all screwed up, and that makes everything even harder.' Will this ever end?" she thought, on the verge of tears.

"We don't allow any of that in here! How many times do I have to tell you?" Jim Hannan asked, grabbing a Kleenex for Jessica from a box next to the scale. He had appeared at her side, taking her by surprise, much as she had startled her husband an hour earlier. She dabbed at a damp spot in the corner of her left eye, trying to smile at the same time.

"Things are looking pretty good," Hannan told her. "His lungs seem to be coming along, thanks to the steroids. If he keeps bopping along like this we're going to have to let him go one of these days, and that would leave us with an empty Isolette."

"I'm sure you'll find a way to fill it," she replied, quickly perking up.

"I guess we will," said Hannan. "Maybe Santa Claus will leave us a seven hundred-gram reindeer. Try to have a Merry Christmas," he said, suddenly serious as he reached for the doorknob. "You two deserve it."

As Hannan rushed out of Room 445 back toward his office, Jessica Durand began gathering up her things. She placed her knitting in the canvas diaper bag she had gotten at an early shower and checked to make sure the tape was running on Stephen's recorder.

"Bye, Jessica," said Susie, as Jessica walked through the tiny office between the sections of the nursery. "Have a nice Christmas if we don't see you before then."

"Merry Christmas to you, too," responded Jessica, smiling. She liked Susie, in part because she was too new to the nursery to be possessive about the babies like the more experienced nurses.

As she passed through the middle section of the nursery Jessica noticed that Arlene and another nurse were checking the equipment on an empty warming table, making sure everything was ready. "What a Christmas present for some couple," thought Jessica as she stripped off her nursery gown. "There must be another baby on the way." She happened to glance at the clock as she pulled on her coat: 1:29. She'd be late getting back to work. As she stepped out into the hallway she was thinking about the job she had returned to about three weeks earlier and how generous her employers were being about allowing her to spend so much time with Stephen. She crossed the hall, rang for the elevator, and was about to cross back for a last peak through the window at Stephen when she heard Mary Anne call, "Coming through please!" and stepped back against the wall just in time to avoid being run down by the Code Pink team, rushing toward the door of 445.

Chapter Six

"What's this?" asked Hannan as he strode over to the warming table in Section B. His hands were busy tying the light-blue gown closed behind his back. He glanced down at the table. "Oh, Jesus," he said softly.

Baby boy Alvarez lay on his back, his chest and grossly distended abdomen rising and falling with each of his sharp, saw-edged cries. His dusky gray-blue color was accentuated by the fact that he had not been bathed before being rushed from the delivery room by the Code Pink team just five minutes earlier, at 1:29. The tan shades had already been lowered across the room's plate-glass windows, protecting both the baby's privacy and the sensibilities of visitors coming to view other infants. There was a term to describe baby boy Alvarez. Not a term found in medical textbooks, but the kind of term picked up after work over a few beers: FLK, funny-looking kid. For baby boy Alvarez simply didn't look right. It wasn't just that he was a 6-pound, 8-ounce baby in a room filled with 2- and 3-pounders. And it wasn't just his clubbed feet and bowed legs, which were obvious. There was something odd about his face. Nothing you could immediately describe. Just something odd.

"This leg's shorter than the other," said Javed, who was examining the baby. He ran his hands over its barrel-shaped abdomen. "I think it's an abdominal mass; it's tense. Can we get a catheter?"

"Get an X-ray! Stat!" Hannan ordered. "Jeees, I wonder if he's got a diaphragmatic hernia [an opening in the diaphragm that would allow bowel to work its way up into the chest]. You hear anything up there?" he asked Javed.

"Yes. I hear sounds," replied the younger man, who was listening to the infant's chest with a stethoscope.

"Is it bowel?"

"I don't know."

"He looks premature on top of it," Hannan observed. It was not the sort of thing an office-based pediatrician would have noticed, for the baby had been delivered by cesarean section at thirty-six weeks, only three weeks shy of his mother's due date.

"I'd put a catheter in," Hannan told Javed, who was being assisted by John Noble, Mary Anne, and Sidney Stevens, one of the unit's respiratory technicians. "But just make sure you put it in the artery or you'll end up someplace funny."

Javed fumbled several times as he tried to insert the tiny plastic tube in the even tinier umbilical artery. The job was complicated by the discovery that baby boy Alvarez had yet another abnormality, a patent urachus. The urachus is a minute connection between bladder and placenta that is supposed to seal itself off long before birth. On rare occasion, however, it doesn't close off, leaving a patent urachus, an opening in the umbilical stump leading to the bladder.

Despite being given supplemental oxygen, baby boy Alvarez was turning a progressively darker shade of blue. "Could we put

him up to one hundred percent oxygen for the time being?"
Javed asked Hannan.

"Put him up to one hundred percent and let's eyeball him and
see where we are," the director replied.

"Somebody call for an X-ray?" asked a young woman who
entered the nursery pushing an infant-sized portable X-ray unit.

"Over here," said Hannan. "Let's see what's in his chest and
get a picture, because I think we're going to have to go to the
respirator with this. Why don't you get your blood gases while
she's getting the picture," he told the lab technician, who was
standing by, waiting to get a sample of the baby's arterial blood
from the now-inserted catheter. As the X-ray technician prepared her equipment, Hannan noticed a new figure in the nursery. A short, pale man with a drooping brown mustache and an
expression to match stood hesitantly just inside the door of the
record area, peering around the corner in an attempt to see what
was being done to the baby on the table—his first child.

"Mr. Alvarez? I'm Dr. Hannan. Why don't we step outside
here?" said the doctor, escorting the father into the hallway.
"The baby has a number of problems," Hannan told Raoul Alvarez, skipping the usual doctor-patient small talk. "We've been
going over the baby and there are what look like some abnormalities of the lower extremities." Alvarez, whose English was a
bit shaky, cocked his head slightly to one side, apparently not
quite sure of what he was being told, but sure of its import. "The
lower limbs seem to have some difficulty with them," Hannan
continued. "In examining the abdomen we've found some lumps
I'm not sure should be there. Most of all your baby's having
difficulty breathing. I don't know why. I don't know whether
he's having difficulty breathing because there's some fluid in the
chest or because there's an abnormality in the chest itself. We're
taking some X-rays now, and as soon as we know something we'll
let you know. Okay?"

"All right. Tank you," replied Raoul Alvarez. Hannan turned

immediately and stepped back into the safety of the nursery. And as soon as the doctor's back disappeared, two women, both speaking in rapid, excited Spanish, descended on Alvarez. They were the grandmothers of the baby on the warming table, and both had come to Metropolitan to be on hand for the joyfully awaited birth of their first grandchild.

"Don't sew that in too tight," Hannan told Javed, who was finishing up the insertion of the umbilical catheter, "because she's going to have to take a wide cone film of the baby. Quite frankly, she's going to have to zip downstairs and tell me whether there's bowel in there or not. He probably has bowel in his chest." The discussion was interrupted by the lab technician, who returned with the results of the first blood workup. "Six point eight pH! Man! A pH of six-eight means he's profoundly acidotic," said Hannan, shaking his head. "Normal is seven point three and it's a log scale," which means that the difference of point 5 between the two lab values really means that one was about twenty times the other. "Goddamn! Boogy! Boogy! Boogy!"

The team worked to get the baby on the respirator, but each time they thought they had the endotracheal tube in, the baby would let out a cry. And a baby can't cry when the tube is properly inserted, because the larynx is immobilized by the tube. The delay in inserting the tube was depriving the baby of oxygen, and not only was his color getting worse, but also he was having trouble with the fluid building up in his lungs. "Suction!" ordered Hannan. "He's really getting raunched." When Sidney Stevens' job of suctioning the baby didn't suit him, Hannan began to call out, "On! Off! On! Off! Come on. Okay, now you've got it . . ." He was interrupted by the X-ray technician, who handed him the first film of baby boy Alvarez's insides.

"*Wooo!*" Hannan exhaled loudly, holding the X-ray up to the fluorescent ceiling light.

"What have you got?" asked Javed, who had finally succeeded in getting the baby on the respirator.

"I don't know," replied Hannan. "A dextrocardia [a rotation of the heart to the right]? I think that might be bowel up there." He stepped over to the light box on the wall and hung the X-ray to view it properly. "He's got a funny, globular heart. It may be a transposition, rather than a dextrocardia. I don't know, but he's got a big right-sided bulge. He may be a hypoplastic [under-developed] left heart with a big right-sided heart. The right side looks like it's got some fluid and the left side's got some crap in there. I don't know what it is. The diaphragm is in just about the worst position, and the catheter's got to go in about two more inches." He pointed at the picture of the catheter with a yellow pencil plucked from behind his left ear.

"He's getting pink," Stevens said, interrupting Hannan's examination of the X-ray.

"Okay," he responded absentmindedly, his thoughts remaining with the image on the light box. "I need some better X-rays," he said. "He's got some really funny bones. He's got flasking. He's got a weird-looking clavicle on this side. That's bizarro! He looks like he's got chondrodystrophy [a malformation of the cartilage]. That's got to be stomach, so that's got to be the right side," he said to Javed, who had joined him at the light box.

"What's that bone on the right side?" asked Javed.

"That's arm."

"No, below that."

"That's weird!" said Hannan, scratching the back of his head. "It could be thymus, but I'm not sure. One way or another, the kid's going to need surgery. Well, I don't know. First we've got to figure out what he's got." He returned to the warming table and began his first careful examination of the body. "Do we have a problem," he said, his voice suddenly soft and even. "You know what that is?" he asked the team, pointing to a few drops of blackish goo oozing from the tip of the baby's penis. "He's passing meconium [prenatal feces] out of there. What do you want to do, guys? We'd better call Bob Albert at home. Frog farts! You ain't supposed to crap through your pecker, kid!" The statement was as much a sign of his increasing puzzlement and frustration as it was typical of his scatalogical and somewhat weird sense of humor.

Hannan stepped around the corner to the phone in the chart area and dialed surgeon Robert Albert's office at St. Francis. "This is Dr. Hannan, Metropolitan Intensive Care, calling for Dr. Robert Albert," he told the page operator who took the call. "Right. Dr. Hannan. Metropolitan." He slammed the receiver down. "You know what we ought to do," he muttered, mostly to himself. "Get a bunch of chemistries, BUN and all that good stuff. Then what I'd love to do," he told Javed and Noble, "is run some dye in there and take a look at his kidneys. But I don't think we can."

"I don't think it's an emergency right now," said Noble.

"I don't think it's an emergency either," his boss told him, "but if I don't see any kidneys in there I know what to do with my ventilator—just turn it off. You don't do a kidney transplant on a kid like this. The other thing to do would be to blow some air in his anus and see where it goes."

"He probably doesn't have an anus," said Noble.

Hannan turned the baby on his side. "Oh, boy. Just a dimple. The kid hasn't got an anus."

"That's interesting," observed Javed.

"Interesting isn't the right word," said Hannan, his tone edged with impatience. The phone rang and he called to whoever was answering it, "I've got Dr. Albert on page!" Albert was the caller, and Hannan quickly outlined all that he thought could be wrong with baby boy Alvarez. Then, almost as soon as he hung up the phone, he took a second call, this one from Dr. Donald Benjamin, the obstetrician who had delivered the baby an hour and a half earlier. "That baby of yours, baby Alvarez or whatever? It's terrible." His voice rose slightly. "It's even worse than you think. The kid has no anus and he's stooling out through his penis and he has cartilagenous anomalies and probably renal anomalies and we've just put him on the ventilator, one hundred percent oxygen, and I think he's probably got transposition or some other cardiac anomaly. I've called a pediatric surgeon, but I don't know exactly what to do. His prospects aren't terribly good. Sure, I think I've heard of him," he said, responding to a question Benjamin asked about a pediatrician the baby's grandmothers wanted brought in for a consult. "I'd be happy to talk to him. I don't even know what problems to tackle. I think the baby's got a lethal constellation of defects, but I'll keep you posted." He hung up once again, this time more gently.

Raoul Alvarez had returned to the nursery and was standing quietly by the warming table, watching as Sidney Stevens adjusted the endotracheal tube. "We're going to be taking some more X-rays shortly," Hannan told him. "In addition to what I told you before, there are some further abnormalities in terms of the baby's intestinal tract as well. The baby's anus, where the baby stools, is absent. The baby's stooling through the penis. You understand?"

"Yes? The penis?" asked the father.

"Yes, the penis, the male organ. The stool that should come out through the anus is coming out through the penis," continued Hannan, "so there's a connection that shouldn't be there between the bowel and the urinary tract. There also is a suspicion in our minds that the upper part of the food tube ends in a blind pouch and that there's a connection between the food tube and the airway, which causes some difficulty breathing. I've asked a pediatric surgeon, Dr. Robert Albert, of St. Francis, to come by. He should be here by four-thirty. He'll chat with you about his findings. I think it's probable there's something wrong with the baby's heart as well. There are many organ systems that are not right, but we'll know more when we get the X-rays."

"So," said Alvarez. "So, what can I say?" He shrugged slightly; his deep brown eyes were filling with tears. "It's stupid to make any . . ."

"That's why we want more information," Hannan interjected. "Dr. Albert is a surgeon and sees many problems and he can tell us if there's anything a surgeon can do."

"What do you think is the reason? We are very healthy," Alvarez told Hannan, as if wishing away the reality of the warming table.

Hannan was about to speak but suddenly seemed to remember that he and the father were not alone. "Why don't we step across the hall where we can sit down?" he said, leading Alvarez the few steps down the corridor to his cubbyhole office.

"I don't know what may have caused this in the past," he began, after establishing his position behind his cluttered desk, "and I don't know what to tell you about future pregnancies. I will, by the time we're finished with this, have some advice as far as how to go about investigating the possibilities of future pregnancies, as well as about what can be done with this baby. But right now, I don't have enough information."

"Of course," the father agreed, leaning forward from his seat on the yellow vinyl couch trapped between filing cabinet and journal-strewn table. "This is very soon."

"I just don't know what could have caused this in the pregnancy," continued Hannan. "It's *extremely*"—he stressed the word—"unlikely that there was any way of knowing about this beforehand, or of being able to say, 'Ah, yes, there was a problem at this time.' With these problems you very often don't know. This is very rare. Perhaps once a year we see something like this. We can't explain it. It's a tragedy."

"What if we took a picture when my wife was pregnant?" asked Alvarez, who, at that point, was blaming his wife's obstetrician for what had happened. They had done everything right, he thought, planned so carefully, behaved so prudently. Maria hadn't taken any medications during her pregnancy. Not even an aspirin! And they had asked Dr. Benjamin whether Maria should have amniocentesis, just to make sure everything was all right. But he had said, "No, Maria, you're only twenty-nine. There's simply no need for it and it would actually involve much more risk than it would be worth." And he had laughed. He had actually laughed!

"It's very doubtful an X-ray would have shown anything," replied Hannan, bringing Alvarez mentally back into the room. "Even something more sophisticated, like ultrasound, probably wouldn't find anything. One of the cruel paradoxes of the kind of defect I think the baby has, is that it's perfectly consistent with the normal function of the baby when it's in the mother, because the placenta is doing the work. And it's only once the baby's born," he continued, "that this kind of heart defect causes a problem. It doesn't cause a problem when the baby's a fetus."

"So the mother keeps it alive?"

"That's right. The baby inside the mother doesn't need much liver. It doesn't need an intestinal tract because it's not feeding. It's not breathing. It's only needed once the baby's born. So what we've done now is put him on a machine to breath for him and put a catheter in the umbilical artery to see how much oxygen he's getting."

"Your only think will be, then, a few hours to see," said Alvarez, whose English was deteriorating along with his hope.

"I want to consult the surgeon to see what, in his experience, can be done," Hannan told him. "I want to know that in his experience and my experience there's no hope. Then the question is: Can we keep the mechanical ventilation going? If there's no hope, it's another question. But to talk specifically about the future isn't appropriate. I will sit down with you again in an hour or so and make some specific plans."

"Forget the legal thing," said Alvarez, who despite his apparent language difficulties, was already way ahead of Hannan in thinking very specifically about the future.

"It has nothing to do with the legal," said Hannan gently. "It has to do with how I'd approach it if it were my baby. It's not sentimental. I want to have all the facts. As long as there's any hope for your baby to have the chance to be normal, I want to explore it. There are still some tests I think we can make. I think it's a very unlikely possibility, but before I say definitely, we need more information. It's early."

"I am very sad," said Alvarez, simply. "My sister, my brother. There is no genetic problem."

"We'll have more information later. Why don't you go down and see your wife now?" said Hannan, rising from his desk chair. "We have to consult and do some more tests. We'll talk later." He placed a hand on the father's shoulder and guided him out of the office. Hannan hurried back to the nursery, expecting Raoul Alvarez to head for the elevator. But Alvarez did not go back to his wife's third-floor room. Instead, after telling his mother and mother-in-law what the doctor had told him, he remained outside the nursery door, awaiting further word from Hannan.

"Hi, Bob," said Hannan as he walked back into the nursery and saw Dr. Robert Albert examining baby boy Alvarez's X-ray.

"That heart. What kind of heart is that?" the surgeon asked.

"Well, it's a little rotated, so I don't know," Hannan told him, "but it looks to me like an egg-shaped heart. It goes along with his gases."

"It's not a diaphragmatic hernia," Albert announced. "The stomach is in the right place, of course. The left side of the chest is very unusual, but . . ."

"I think there's some chondrodystrophy," said Hannan, and the surgeon agreed. After learning what he could from the one, poor-quality X-ray, Albert stepped over to the warming table and examined baby boy Alvarez. His hands moved quickly—poking here, squeezing there. It was over in less than two minutes.

"Well, the imperforated anus isn't life-threatening for the moment. There's no esophegeal atresia, and the heart lesion is the limiting factor."

"So I called the wrong specialist?"

"If the cardiac lesion can't be dealt with, there's no point in my doing anything with the other problems," Albert told him.

"The chain of logic argues that if surgery can't help the

heart . . ." Hannan paused. "Let's set up a cardiogram and see
what that looks like. And I guess I better give Arnie a call and
have him come take a look at the kid." Hannan immediately
placed a call to pediatric cardiologist Arnold Greenberg at St.
Francis and stepped out in the hall to update Raoul Alvarez.

"It's not terribly helpful," he told the anxious father. "There
are still a couple of things that are a distinct possibility, including a couple that are inoperable. One major possibility is that the
left side of the baby's heart, the part that pumps the blood to the
whole body, not just the lungs, is underdeveloped. That really
would be inoperable. I think maybe that's just the right side of
the heart that we're seeing and it's gotten big to compensate for
the left side. Also, just now we've had to make a rather drastic
change in the ventilator. You saw the baby get very blue and also
gray and mottled-looking. This sometimes happens as this part of
the . . ."

Alvarez interupted him. "You have to do all you can, but . . ."
He was stopped by tears.

"What do you think?" Hannan asked.

"If he lives, he's going to suffer."

"You're welcome to stay," said Hannan, his eyes focusing on
the tips of his desert boots.

"It was our first baby," the father said, tears streaming down
his cheeks.

"What can I say?" the neonatologist asked quietly. He had
been through this scene dozens of times, and somehow it never
surprised him that each was as difficult as the one before.

"You still want to keep trying," Alvarez asked Hannan. It was
as much a statement as a question.

"I'll keep going on like this until the cardiologist talks to us,"
Hannan replied. "There's not much more I can do."

"I don't want the baby to suffer," the father told him.

"Neither do I," Hannan said slowly.

Alvarez turned away from the doctor and walked over to the
elevators. He pressed the down button and then leaned against

the wall, his face buried in the crook of his gowned arm, his body shaking slightly. Knowing there was nothing more he could do, Hannan returned to Albert in the nursery.

"I've arranged to take some blood back with me when I go," Albert told Hannan when the neonatologist returned to the nursery. "I'll drop it off with Jack O'Connell [the chief of genetics at St. Francis]. That may be the most important thing now," said Albert. "By the way, Arnie has a patient who can be transferred out of the nursery over there so we can get baby Alvarez in."

"I really like Arnie," said Hannan. "He's a good cardiologist. But I don't think there's much he's going to be able to tell us, unless he's willing to do echo cardiography [which uses sound waves to create a picture of the heart]. But as I told him over the phone, the landmarks may be so disturbed that he won't know what to do. What he's going to have to do is figure out whether there's enough of a chance and whether he can do anything. That's the way it's going to stack up. See, a cardiogram doesn't look too good diagnostically. The baby's got a lot of right-sided force and not much left side. That could either be transposition, or hypoplastic left heart. Arnie, with his expertise, may be able to look at it and say, 'Ya, it's hypoplastic left heart.' But even then it may be operable. He may be able to say that it's nonoperable, but he may not be able to say with any certainty that it is. And that's going to be the problem: How's he going to weigh one against the other? But you feel fairly—I don't want to use the word optimistic—you feel that there's a reasonable chance for the other anomalies?" Hannan asked his colleague.

"Yeah, they certainly are not life-threatening."

"They're not inoperable?"

"They're operable."

"What we don't know," said Hannan, "is if there's anything in the kidneys. I tried to palpate the kidneys and I just couldn't get anything."

"It's doughy on both sides," said Albert.

"It felt like big dilated ureters, which you would expect. He just put out a little bit of urine mixed with meconium," Hannan told Albert.

"That's encouraging," said the surgeon, who then sat down to write his notes into the baby's chart. After listing ten possible anomalies he wrote: "Problems are surgically correctable and not life-threatening at this time. If cardiac lesion does not curtail survival, child needs lap for colostomy and closure of patent urachus."

It was only 4:30, but Hannan was beginning to drag as he walked back to his office, where he immediately flopped into his chair and flung one leg across the desk. Almost simultaneously Karen Fitzgerald tapped on the door and stuck her head into the office. Hannan waved her in.

"Oh, that shit in there," exhaled Hannan as Fitzgerald plopped down on the couch. "You feel sorry for another human being. I don't know what to do. If the kid has a lethal defect, you can be positive the kid's going to die. But you come to that little thread. Now how far out on that thread do you go? I keep stringing it out to Arnie. I know what Arnie's going to say; he's going to say, 'Oh ya, we can ship him over.' I'm going to get waffles; that's what I'm going to get."

"So do we just give him the baby and let him take it from there?" asked Fitzgerald, who in her two months at Lying-In had never had to deal with a baby in as bad shape as baby boy Alvarez. Fitzgerald was well aware of Hannan's belief and policy that a baby should be transferred to another facility only for care that couldn't be provided at Lying-In and should be returned to Lying-In once that care was provided. But this, the resident thought, had to be a special situation.

"No," Hannan explained, "the only thing special about the case is the seriousness of the baby's condition, and that would not affect the more basic question of who would bear ultimate responsibility for the baby's care. Arnie and I will just talk about it," said Hannan, "like I did with Bob. If Bob had said something outrageous, then it's my baby and my decision to make. Arnie's a pretty rational guy. He'll give me odds and he'll give me a more valuable opinion than I could make for myself as far as the possible problems go. Then I'll have to weigh them."

"You said it might be a duct. Why?" the young woman asked.

"A variety of cardiac lesions are duct-dependent," Hannan told her. "That means that all the systemic flow is going through the patent ductus. As the patent ductus closes, it's like putting a ligature around your aorta and closing off the flow. The ductus closes as the oxygen goes up. So as you improve them, their oxygen goes up but they start getting worse. The oscillations of getting better and getting worse get narrower and narrower and the slope is down until they just peel off.

"I can shove some prostaglandin in and open the ductus up," Hannan told the resident, who was leaning forward, listening intently as he rambled on, "but that doesn't always work. That's the pisser about this business: There's always one more little thing that you might try, one more little thing that you could do, one more little exercise. It's the thing people don't understand. Talk about extraordinary care, or heroic care—it's impossible in many instances to differentiate. There's always one more little thing. Clearly what we're doing is heroic. Now, if I were to go in there and shove a catheter up through his aorta, through his ductus into his heart, and maneuver it, I could perfuse him downstream for a while. I could give him something to open up his pulmonary system. There're always a few things. Every once in a while you get a kid who turns into wet tissue paper and falls apart. But most of the time there's always one other little thing you can do, and at some point you've got to stop. And that's not a clear line most of the time. It's dirty."

"But to keep doing those things don't you have to have a reason?" Fitzgerald asked. "Doesn't there have to be something at the other end?"

"It's never that clear, you see? There's always a chance. Suppose Arnie comes in and says there's a three-and-one-half percent chance it's an operable cardiac defect. Bob has said, 'Well, ya, I don't know about his kidneys'—which is a great big fuzzy gray cloud—'but we can do this, and we can do this, and he's got about a thirty percent chance of survival.' And we haven't even said a word about his head!" exclaimed Hannan, his voice rising. "Suppose we do all this, and whittle on him, and he's got a big cyst sitting right in the middle of his gourd? I haven't asked that. I just say let's look at what we can see."

"What are the odds he has a major neurological anomaly?"

"If he had a cleft palate then I'd try to light him up and see if his head glows. I ought to go in there and do that."

Despite having heard of such procedures, Fitzgerald still cringed slightly every time she thought about the idea of lighting an infant's head up like a jack-o-lantern. She quickly changed the subject by asking Hannan what Raoul Alvarez really meant when he said in one breath that he didn't want his baby to suffer and then in the next said he wanted the doctors to do all they could.

"He's saying just that and nothing more. I can't make anything more of it or it becomes my personal opinion. In this business I've learned that what they're telling you is the truth," Hannan told her, fiddling nervously with one of his yellow pencils. "He wants me to do what I think is best, to go as far as I think I can. He's giving me a lot of trust. He doesn't want the child to suffer. I don't want the child to suffer either. The whole thing about suffering needlessly becomes totally irrelevant. What's needless?" he rhetorically asked the young woman. "I can't start playing those games. I can't say, 'Well, he really wants this, or he really wants that.' That's a really good way to make an error.

"If I make a decision," Hannan continued, "I'm going to tell him, 'If this were my child,' or however you want to phrase it. Now if he says, 'No, you can't stop trying!' then I can't. That's it. But sometimes you get parents who say, 'Why don't you let him go? You really ought to let him go. He's got this and he's got that.' Sometimes they argue against stopping. But often they don't. They say, 'Why don't you let him rest?' And I'll say, 'Because there is still some possibility and I'd like to exhaust it.'

"Once you stop, it's irrevocable. It all then becomes cocktail party talk and opinion. It's mathematically an entirely different ballgame. You see, all this has numbers on it: theory, chances, odds, even if it's one percent or point one percent or a millionth of a percent. It's still in numerical sequence. As soon as you start talking about life and death, it's like talking about boys and girls: It's yes or no; it's absolute. So why the hurry to decide? The only reason is the baby may be suffering. Well, who the hell knows? If they're really worried about that I can dope the kid up so he doesn't look like he's suffering. I can give him curare and he won't move. Or I can give him morphine and he won't move. That don't make no difference.

"It's funny," Hannan told Fitzgerald, who had been sitting speechless through his discourse, "but I'd like to have an ethicist here going through this like you are, because they're really good at discussion. They're always good after the fact, and with cocktail party talk. They have a lot of answers and a lot of questions and they can turn you upside down and inside out. But I never notice them getting out on the firing line. I mean, what would an ethicist do with that question in there?" he asked, gesturing across the hall toward the nursery. "I don't want the baby to suffer, but I want him to have every chance. I don't know, it's interesting—like how many angels can dance on the head of a pin? It makes people too uncomfortable to deal with it. It makes me uncomfortable and I *have to* deal with it."

"How do you deal with the relatives?" asked Fitzgerald, who was, herself, growing uncomfortable dealing with the subject under discussion, and who was also genuinely interested in knowing how Hannan was handling two semihysterical grand-mothers in the hallway.

"Ignore them," was the answer. "You've got to do it that way. Otherwise you can get trapped in a power struggle without even realizing it. The mother-in-law, the mother, who's the first one to talk to the doctor and take the information down to the room? You don't need that. I tend to ignore them or give them simple, factual, answers. I've got enough problems now. I'm going to have to go down and deal with the wife." Hannan slapped the palms of both hands down on his desk and gestured with his head toward the door. Karen Fitzgerald pulled herself up off the couch and left the office. Hannan followed her down the hall into the nursery.

"That's the weirdest heart I've ever seen," cardiologist Arnold Greenberg was saying to himself as Hannan walked up to him. Greenberg, like Robert Albert before him, was standing in front of the light box, transfixed by the translucent black-and-white image of baby boy Alvarez's internal organs.

"What do you think?" Hannan asked.

"I think it's cyanotic heart disease," Greenberg told him.

"Do you think it's hypoplastic left heart, on the basis of the cardiogram?"

"I think there are some left ventricular forces, but that doesn't mean anything. I don't think you can tell anything with echo with this heart. It's in such an unusual position. And you know what's so unusual about it? All vascularity is on the left and there's nothing on the right. So he might very well have no right pulmonary artery, or something along those lines."

"What's that?" asked Hannan, pointing to a spot on the X-ray.

"I don't know," the cardiologist admitted.

"Left side of the heart?"

"No, it's too big, unless it's a huge truncus. But it's arching up so high."

"What do you think his chances of having an operable lesion are?" Hannan came to the point.

"I have no idea," said Arnold Greenberg, the man Hannan had called for help.

"When do you want to transfer him?"

"If they want to do something about him," Greenberg replied. "The thing that I'd be concerned about is whether or not he could tolerate the dye from angiography." He shook his head. "That's the weirdest heart I've ever seen, with the vascularity all on the left."

"You're not making me feel any better," said Hannan.

"Nobody could tell you what this is," Greenberg responded. "They could only guess. I mean, statistically, it's transposition. But I just don't know. There's no way I can tell. If it's transposition, then he's got selective pulmonary stenosis of the right pulmonary artery because there's nothing going there and this is all increased vascularity."

"Then the pulmonary flow could be normal?"

"It could be," said Greenberg, who then laid out several other possibilities for Hannan and concluded by asking, "The parents want to go, right?"

"The parents don't want the kid to suffer; they want us to do what we can."

"He's got an anal atresia; we don't know the status of his GI system, but statistically . . ."

"He's got doughy masses in his flanks which suggest dilated ureters," Hannan interrupted him.

"That's going to affect his catheterization," Greenberg told him, "because if I cath him and he doesn't excrete the dye, the only way I can make the diagnosis is angiographically, and he's going to die from the procedure."

"He's put out a little bit of urine mixed with meconium through his penis. That's a cloaca he's got there," guessed Hannan, who had no way of knowing it was his most accurate bit of diagnostic speculation yet. "Let's look at it this way: If he dies in the procedure, that's okay, if there's a chance that we can find something that you can do something with. When I say a chance, I mean if it's reasonable that you can find something operable."

"Well . . ."

"You tell me and I can take it from here. If you say the odds of the cath, plus finding anything, is remote, I can sell the folks on that and we'll just let the kid stay here and snuff," Hannan said, stating the facts with the brutal simplicity that sometimes characterized his assessment of situations. "Bob isn't super-gungho. What he's saying, in honesty, is that if you think he has a cardiac problem that's reparable, then he's willing to try the others."

"The problem is, if it's a dextraversion with an aplastic left heart, then his left ventrical is going to be the anterior ventrical and I'm not going to be able to echo it," said Greenberg, thinking out loud. "But being cyanotic, and with a dextraversion, it's more than likely he's got pulmonary atresia. I think it's worth a chance."

"Okay," said Hannan, who suddenly looked relaxed for the first time since baby boy Alvarez had been brought into the nursery four hours earlier. "I'll tell the folks. At least we've got a trump card there. That's the best news I've heard all day!"

"I'd say there's about a twenty-five percent chance he'll die on the cath table," Greenberg added, "but there's a one hundred percent chance he'll die if he stays here."

But as far as Hannan was concerned, the problem with baby boy Alvarez was solved. "How's the kid with meconium?" he asked a passing nurse, turning his attention immediately to the regular business of the nursery and a baby who was a long-term resident.

As Arnold Greenberg made the necessary arrangements for the transfer of the Alvarez baby—assembling his catheterization team, reserving the cath room, alerting the St. Francis nursery that he would need a respirator and warming table, and calling for the transfer team—Hannan walked downstairs to Room 345 to give the news to Maria and Raoul Alvarez. His presentation to them, made after asking the grandmothers to leave the room, was brief and to the point. If the baby stayed at Metropolitan, he would die; at least Hannan thought he would. If he were transferred, there was about a 25 percent chance he would die in the ambulance and at least a 25 percent chance he would die during the catheterization—and that was just a diagnostic procedure to determine whether surgery could do him any good.

It didn't take Maria Alvarez any time at all to make her decision. "You say it is not a one hundred percent chance, not even a fifty percent chance the baby will live if you take him to St. Francis. If the baby cannot live, why make an operation and make him suffer? So if the baby has to die, he will die in the same place where he is born." She looked at the doctor, standing at the foot of her bed, and tried to guess what he was thinking. Did he think her cruel, a beast who cared nothing for her baby? Or did he understand? Could he understand why a mother would rather have her new baby die than have it suffer, have it live as half a person?

"All right," Hannan said, answering her unasked questions. "We'll do what we can to make your baby comfortable. We'll see how it goes tonight, and I'll come down in the morning and we can talk about where to go from here. I just want you to know one thing: If I were in your position, I'd make the decision you just made."

"Thank you, Doctor Hannan. And thank you for being honest with me. Can you tell me one thing?" the mother asked, still a bit groggy from the anesthesia given her for her cesarean delivery. "Is my baby in pain?"

"I can't really tell you," Hannan replied, honestly. "But if you want me to I can give the baby some morphine. Then I can assure you he won't be suffering."

"Please."

"I'll be back to see you later," said Hannan. He turned and left the room. "Goddamn!" he thought as he walked down the hall, shaking his head in amazement. "That is one together lady!"

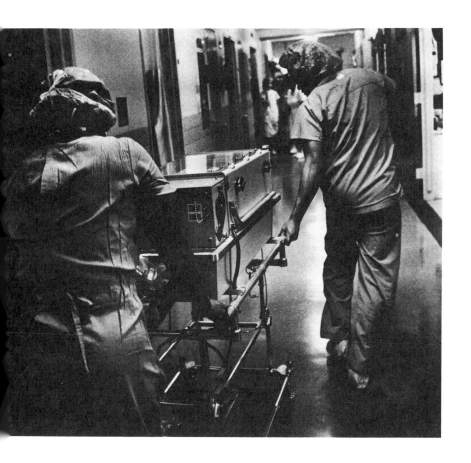

"The elevator doors opened at the fourth floor and the infant transporter was rolled down the hall with Javed pulling and the women pushing and guiding it. The transporter contains a respirator; air compressor and blender; oxygen supply; its own electrical supply; lights; monitors for heart, respiration, and central venous pressure; and a heating element over the top in a clear plastic cover, similar to the defroster unit in the windshield of a 747 jet. The baby can be observed through the radiant heating element, and the cover can be slid out of the way enough for the team to reach under the edge to work on the baby and, at the same time, keep the baby warm."

The infants and grownups in these photographs are not those described in the book.

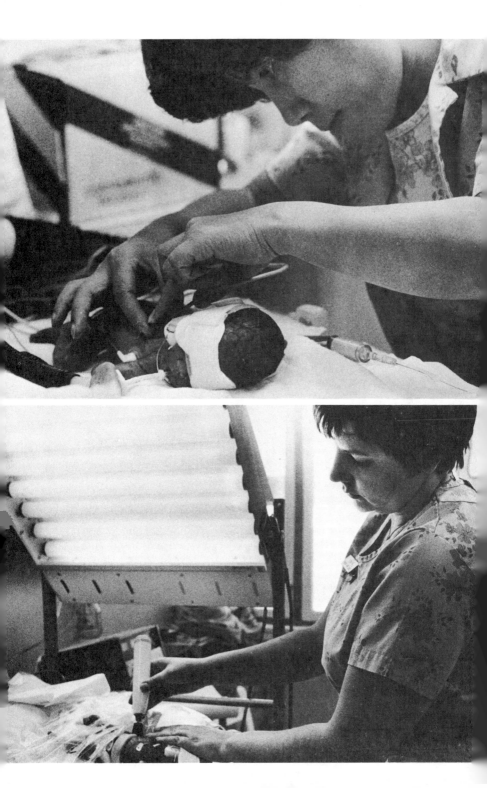

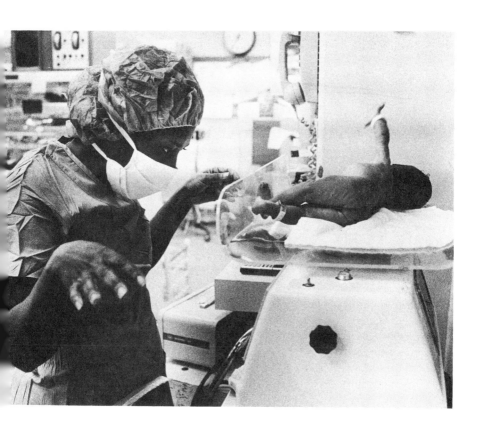

"Each baby in the nursery had a primary nurse—one person responsible for writing nursing orders and overseeing nursing care. Even though the primary nurse is only on one eight-hour shift in a twenty-four-hour day, the system also guarantees some continuity of nursing care and assures the parents that one person knows what's happening to their baby on a minute-by-minute basis.

"Like the other ICN nurses, Evie's day revolved around the one or two babies in her charge. Because Sam Fisher was on a respirator, he was receiving one-to-one nursing care—he was Evie's sole responsibility. While she would help out with other babies when she had a free minute, Sam always came first. Unlike the unit nurse in a general hospital, the twenty-four-year-old woman spent all but her lunch hour within about ten feet of her patient, and most of the eight-hour-shift she was beside his warming table suctioning secretions from his lungs and throat, responding to monitor alarms, changing diapers the size of tiny sanitary napkins, sterilizing equipment for future use, and administering medications through Sam's IVs."

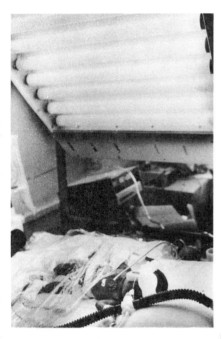

"The first time I saw my one-day-old baby, lying in her incubator in the Intensive Care Nursery, an incredible sadness overwhelmed me. Three-pound Sarah Elizabeth, born in the twenty-eighth week of my pregnancy, looked more like a baby kitten than a baby human, her tiny red body and bony limbs covered with fuzzy dark hair. She had an IV inserted in her leg and she was hooked up to heart and respiration monitors by a maze of wires attached to plastic circles glued to her chest and leg.

"I found it difficult to identify with the tiny creature in the glass box; to acknowledge her as my child. I felt I had somehow failed her, causing her to be born into a world she wasn't ready for, a world of bright lights and loud noises, a world that forced her to breathe, where people handled her and inserted tubes down her throat and stuck needles into her—a world so different from the peaceful, warm, dark, wet place inside me which she was entitled to call home for at least two more months."

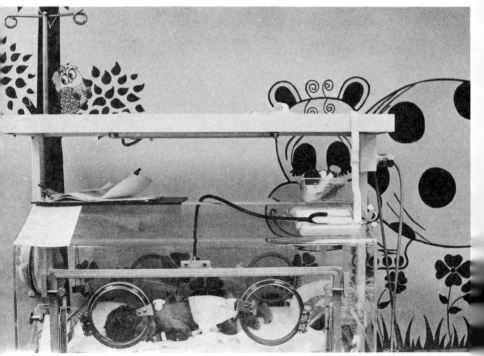

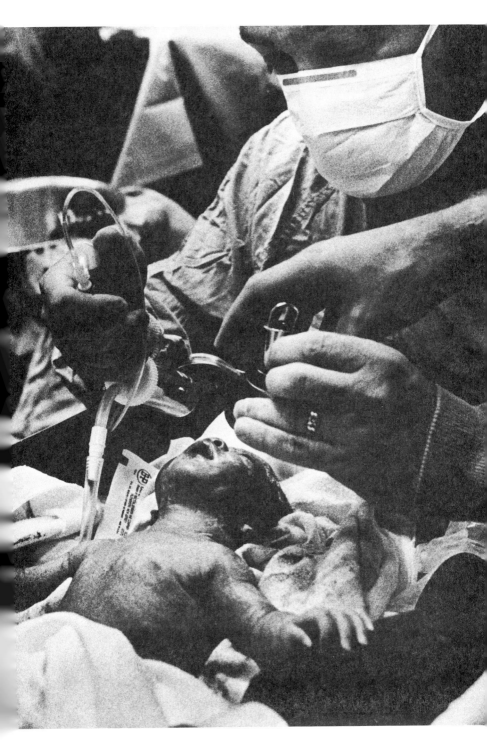

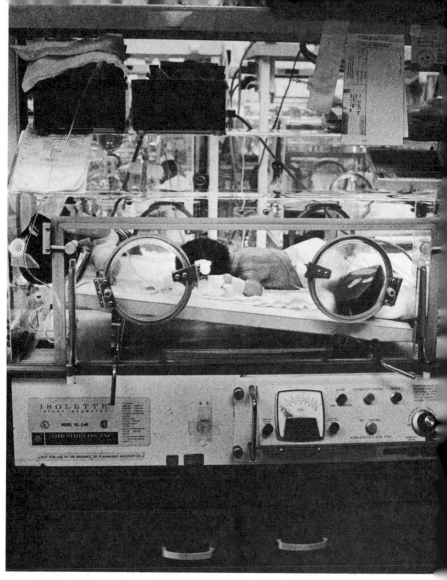

"I'd never seen anything so small, or felt such a wrenching in my stomach. I didn't think I could ever feel so many conflicting emotions as I did then. I just wanted to gather you up in my arms and take you out of there! You were surrounded by all this machinery, with these huge hands and tubes all over you. Your chest was the only thing moving, and that seemed so artificial. You looked like a horse with a bit with that Logan bar. You were just overwhelmed by all that paraphernalia, and I felt preempted. Maybe that's the wrong word, but I was definitely put on the sidelines. There was nothing I could do for you."

Chapter Seven

"Some things never get any easier," Jim Hannan thought as he sat at his desk, chewing on a stale ham and cheese sandwich from the first-floor vending machine as he sorted through the day's mail. "If I'm in this business another hundred years I'll never get used to dealing with that shit with mothers." In over a decade in ICNs he'd seen enough deformity and death to accept it as a part of life. What he would never get used to, however, was having to work with parents in those situations. He could do it; he'd have gone into general pediatrics long ago if he couldn't have handled it. But he'd never be comfortable with it.

Hannan knew he was good at his job. One of the best. Some of his trouble dealing with certain elements of the city's medical community stemmed, in fact, from his refusal ever to pull punches, and from his insistence on always showing just how much he knew or what his nursery could accomplish, even if it meant making other physicians look inept. But that didn't mean he wasn't aware of his own limitations, and the limitations of the science of newborn medicine. He would often remind John Noble that saving babies weighing no more than four average-size tangerines is "a lot like goose hunting: You have to do everything right and *then* get lucky." Of course, every time he said that, he would remember with great clarity the first time he did everything exactly wrong—and then got lucky.

It was a cold, wet, windy, early spring night in 1966, the kind of night that can make even the dark corridors of Boston Lying-In Hospital seem warm and friendly. It was shortly after 1 A.M., and first-year pediatric resident Jim Hannan was already in the second-floor nursery, having been summoned about twenty minutes earlier to restart an IV for one of the babies. He had finished his work and kidded with the nurses for a few minutes and was about to return to the first-floor dorm room used by the on-call residents when the page system crackled again: "Pediatric on call. Please report to DR 1. Stat!"

"Shit," thought Hannan, "there goes the night."

He sprinted up the two flights of stairs to the delivery suites on the fourth floor and, changing gowns at the door, rushed into Delivery Room 1. The charge up the stairs cleared his head, which had been a bit fogged after seventeen hours on duty. And the scene that greeted him as he stood in the doorway, his heart still pounding from the run, would remain with him forever. In the center of the room, beneath the bank of overhead surgical lights, a woman lay asleep on the delivery table, a nurse-anesthetist monitoring her gases. To the right of the woman's feet the anesthesiologist, his back to Hannan, was bent over a small table, frantically working on a baby Hannan could not see. The obstetrician, too, hovered over the little table, darting back and forth between his adult and newborn patients. "Where's that damn pediatrician?!" the obstetrician asked—frantically, Hannan thought—as the resident entered the room.

"You rang?" Hannan asked, announcing his presence.

"Thank God you're here!" said the obstetrician, a man Hannan knew by reputation rather than experience. "We've got an Apgar of 1, swollen belly, the baby's cyanotic, and . . ."

"Term?" Hannan asked, as he took his place at the table.

"About thirty-six weeks," said the obstetrician, who had returned to the baby's mother.

The infant lay on her back on the table as the anesthesiologist worked to get an endotracheal tube into her. She was, as the OB had said, quite blue. Hannan immediately began helping the anesthesiologist with the tube, but, as he would recall later, "the belly kept getting in the way." Indeed, the baby's obviously distended abdomen was her most prominent feature. With the confidence of someone who doesn't really know what he's doing and therefore isn't afraid to do it wrong, Hannan decided that the first thing he had to do was get the belly out of the way so he could work on the baby more easilly. So he called for a needle and proceeded to draw 100 milliliters, about 3.3 ounces, of fluid from the baby's abdomen, immediately reducing its weight by three percent. He had never seen a baby like this before, but from what he *had* seen, he guessed the baby was suffering from some sort of heart failure. And since he had been taught that heart failure should be treated with digitalis, Hannan gave the baby digitalis. Then, after a quick check with the obstetrician, the young resident screamed for 100 milliliters of Rh negative blood, which he pumped into the baby. Between the blood and the oxygen provided by the anesthesiologist, the infant's color quickly changed from blue to pink. Hannan ordered the baby taken to the Intensive Care Nursery, and an hour later the baby was given an exchange transfusion, a complete replacement of her blood, to combat the incompatibility between her blood type and that of her mother.

It wasn't until hours later, when he had a chance to check one of his textbooks, that Jim Hannan learned what he had done. It became obvious from a quick rereading of the proper section of the text that Sara Winthrop was a hydropic baby. And, according to the latest literature, 99.9 percent of all babies with hydrops die in the delivery room. The condition, which most often results from an Rh incompatibility between infant and mother eventually causes the tissues of the body to absorb fluid from the lungs. The infant becomes bloated as fluid builds up around the heart and in the lungs, which leads to congestive heart failure. The only bits of advice the text offered were to avoid using digitalis and to give the baby an immediate exchange transfusion. Nowhere did it mention first reducing the amount of fluid in the baby's overloaded system.

Hannan would learn a few years later that while he had been lucky with Sara, he had not, despite the text, done the wrong thing. For each time in the next decade that he was called to the delivery room for a hydrops baby, Hannan did what he had done that night at Boston Lying-In. And each time the baby lived to reach the nursery. Sara Winthrop did beautifully despite her rocky start. By the age of seven she was tested as having an IQ of 130, was taking riding and piano lessons, and was doing well in school. The other two hydrops babies Hannan saved didn't fare as well. One, as he told John Noble, died a few weeks later of hyaline membrane disease. But that baby had been a victim of immaturity, rather than the Rh problem. The third, he told the Fellow as the two were driving north along I-270 for a morning of autumn fishing, was killed by a nurse.

"Killed by a who?" asked Noble.

"A nurse. You know them, the ladies in white. Well, green or floral prints actually." Hannan glanced over at Noble out of the corner of his right eye, keeping his left on the road the Datsun Z was covering at about eighty-five miles per hour.

"I know what a nurse is. But how did a nurse kill the baby?"

"Loaded him up with salt. It was back in the days when we were still mixing our own IV solutions in that area by the sink. Well, one of the nurses put too much sodium in the bag and then the primary nurse hung it. The kid arrested and we couldn't do a damn thing. I had an idea what might have happened, and when

the blood work came back it was confirmed: the kid had a sodium of two-twelve."

"Jesus. What happened?"

"It was a bitch. The really awful part about it was the kid was
doing really well. The hydrops wasn't a problem and he had had
some hyaline membrane disease but we'd licked that. It really
looked like everything was going to work out. To top it all off,
the father's brother was a pediatrician."

"What did you tell the parents?" Noble asked, wondering
what he'd do in a similar situation.

"I told the mother. What else could I do? I went down to her
room and said, 'I'm afraid I have some very bad news.' I told her
that, as she knew, things had been going quite well, but there'd
been an accident. I just said flat out that too much sodium had
been put in an IV solution and the baby had died."

"She really go off the wall?"

"No. Just the opposite, quite frankly. She just sort of looked at
me for a minute, and then said something about how it must
have been God's will. Said the baby was obviously not meant to
live, and it was a miracle it had ever gotten out of the delivery
room, and she was grateful for all we'd done for the kid."

"And that was that?"

"That, as they say, was that. Of course Norman Rogers went
absolutely crazy."

"Was he the private pediatrician for the kid?" Noble asked.

"Yeah. He just went bonkers when he found out I'd told the
mother. 'Are you crazy?! What in hell did you do that for?!
You're gonna get sued! I'm gonna get sued! The hospital's gonna
get sued! You shouldn't have told her!' You know Norman."

"Oh yes," said Noble, who not only knew Rogers but also had
had his own run-ins with him and knew of Hannan's long-stand-
ing feud with the physician. "What did you tell him?"

"I said, 'Look, Norm, what the hell would you expect me to
do? In the first place, you can't cover up something like this. It'll

come out at the post mortem. On top of that, the mother's brother-in-law is a doctor, and how long do you think it'll be before he starts asking questions? And in the second place, I just don't operate that way. If I make a mistake, or someone working for me makes a mistake, that's that. A mistake has been made.' And that," Hannan told his companion, "was the begining of my trouble with Norm. Look at that, will you," he said, ending the discussion, "isn't that a pretty sight? It's my favorite view up here."

The car had just crested a hill a few miles south of Frederick, Maryland. The town of Frederick was spread out below them in the distance. To the left, the hills rolled off in the direction of Harpers Ferry, West Virginia, and the mountains beyond. To their right they could see more of the northern Maryland countryside. It was a bright, crystal-clear, early October day, and the deep, cloudless blue of the sky was a perfect backdrop for the golden stubble of the surrounding fields and yellows, reds, oranges, browns, and greens of the fall foliage. Hannan often escaped for a half-day, or occasionally an entire day, of fishing or bird hunting, sports that provided him with a complete release from the tensions and problems of the nursery. But they were two sports he pursued with the same precision, seriousness, and attention to detail with which he ran the nursery. Noble had asked to join Hannan on one of his early-morning expeditions, and Hannan had been happy to have him come along. He was a bit chagrined, however, when he arrived at Noble's house shortly before dawn and the Fellow stumbled out without either hip or chest waders. "Hell, John, you ain't gonna catch nothin' if you can't get in the water," Hannan had reprimanded him.

"Oh, I'm in great shape," Noble responded, as he placed his single bag of gear in the back of the car crammed with graphite and bamboo fly rods, tackle boxes, chest waders, hip waders, and other equipment.

"Yeah, great. You know that water's cold. Summer's over, fella."

"I know. That's why I brought these," said Noble, who reached into his canvas sack and pulled out two thirty-five-gallon green plastic trash bags.

"Holy shit! You're planning on catching one mighty big fish," said Hannan.

"Fish? I'm gonna wear these on my feet. I'll just wrap them with waterproof tape and I'm all set," said Noble, laughing.

"Jesus! You're gonna get me thrown out of the woods by Smokey the Bear," Hannan told him. "Anybody sees you wearing those things and you're with me, I'm going to be the laughing stock of the great outdoors from here to Bangor! Garbage bags? What are you planning to do? Get a job with Woodsy Owl cleaning up the forest?" Hannan continued ribbing Noble for about 10 miles, but the ribbing was good-natured and served to break down much of the student-teacher, boss-worker reserve that existed back in the nursery. In fact, by the time they were halfway to Harpers Ferry, where they planned to fish just below the confluence of the Potomac and Shenandoah rivers, Noble decided to take a chance on trying to find out more about what made his boss tick, a question that had fascinated him ever since his first interview with Hannan. He had never met anyone with so many contrasting facets—so charming and kind with the parents of the babies he cared for, yet so rough and uncompromising on those who worked for and with him; so obviously intelligent and perceptive, yet unwilling to compromise or pull his verbal punches, even when failing to do so might mean losing whatever chance he might have of reaching a particular goal. He knew Hannan as a man totally absorbed in the scientific minutiae of the nursery at 11 A.M. who, by noon, could be talking like a truck driver over his car's CB, headed for the nearest trout stream.

"What got you started?" Noble asked Hannan.

"Fishing?"

"No. I mean in medicine. I know it may sound like a dumb question, but I'm always curious about how people get into this business."

"I guess it was two things: My mother was a nurse, and I always wanted to do something using my mind and my hands," Hannan told him. "I was in and out of trouble a lot," he told Noble, "stealing cars and hubcaps, beating people up and getting beaten up." Hannan grew up on the wrong side of the tracks in Yonkers, New York. His mother was the first high school graduate on either side of the family, and his father was a power company lineman, and later foreman, with a seventh-grade education and a deep love of the outdoors. "He used to hunt and fish and talk about when he was growing up," Hannan told Noble, attempting to explain his own love of woods and stream. "My aunt and uncle had a place out in Ardsley. It's a grubby suburb now but it was real country then. There were deer and trout and pheasant. Up until the time I was about eight we could ride the trolley, then a bus, out there. My aunt and uncle still own the place; it's stuck between two housing developments and the stream is filthy. Jesus, I took my older kids out there once and was telling them about the pheasant and deer and all. Bob just looked around, said 'Sure, Dad,' gave me one of these 'bullshit' whistles, and spun his finger around like I'm nuts."

"You went through the public schools there?" asked Noble.

"Yep. I went to Hawthorne Junior High with Fred Morris, in fact—until his parents pulled him out and put him in private school."

"You mean Fred Morris at Children's? The cardiovascular surgeon, Fred Morris?"

"The same one. I'd been in town for three years before I realized it was him. I'd even talked to him on the phone half a dozen times for God's sake, and all of a sudden it dawned on me that Fred was Fred."

"What straightened you out, if you were such a juvenile delinquent?" asked Noble. "Not that you're all that straightened out now."

"I guess the fact that there were a few teachers who took a special interest in me. I had a sixth-grade teacher who kept pushing me all the time. She just wouldn't take second-best. Every Goddamn thing I gave her, she'd hand back to me and say, 'You can do better than this. Now take this back and do it over until you know it's as good as it can be.' Jesus! I'd get pissed at her. But I'd do it. And she was right. Because the second time I'd always do better. I had a couple teachers like that. They'd see how well I tested and then they just wouldn't accept any crap from me. And then there was Mr. Jacobson."

"Jacobson? Who was he, an advisor?"

"No. Jacobson was an assistant principal at Yonkers High. One Thursday afternoon in my junior year he stopped me in the hall and asked whether I was planning to take the Regents exams that Saturday—New York has this statewide college scholarship system, and you can qualify by scoring well on this exam they give you in your junior year. Well, I told him I wasn't going to waste my time, and I'll never forget what he told me."

"What?" Noble asked. "Did he give you the you'll-regret-not-going-to-college-it'll-change-your-life lecture?"

"No. He said, 'If I don't see you in that exam room Saturday I'll break your arm.' And he meant it. He was an ex-Marine, but not very ex. A really bad dude. We'd tangled enough before for me to know that he didn't say things lightly. So I took the exam and got the twelfth of thirteen full Regents scholarships. I graduated from high school fiftieth out of three hundred, made the National Honor Society, and ended up in Columbia on a full scholarship.

"Even though I wanted to be a doctor I took some weird things in college," he continued, as he drove across the rolling hills toward Harpers Ferry. "I took sociology, a lot of statistics, and some really funny things, too, like architecture." Hannan spent his summers working in a hospital on Cape Cod, where he met the girl who was to become his first wife, a doctor's daughter. They were married at the end of his junior year and moved into his parents' home in Yonkers. A husband and soon a father, Hannan had to work two jobs during his senior year at Columbia, one of them as a night clerk in what he described to Noble as a "grade-Z hotel. You know the kind of place. A guy would come in with some honey and say, 'Me and my wife want a room.' I'd say, 'Okay,' and then he'd turn to her and say, 'Hey, babe, what kind of cigarettes do you smoke?' That kind of place."

Hannan was accepted at Boston University Medical School and, following his graduation from Columbia, headed off with his wife to Cape Cod for a summer of work "in a cranberry bog for one dollar an hour—me and the Puerto Rican indentured servants. I did learn how to throw an axe, though. I can still bury an axe in a tree at twenty paces. Learned it from the Puerto Ricans," he told Noble. Hannan's father-in-law lent him the money for his first year of medical school but died that year, leaving his son-in-law heading into the second year of med school ninth in his class with $15 in his pocket.

"How did you make it?" Noble asked, fascinated by this side of Hannan he had never seen before.

"There was a woman in the Registrar's office, Linda Nixon was her name, who found me some money. And I got the job of class projectionist: I was the one who had to stay awake through my second, third, and fourth years of medical school." Hannan worked up to five jobs at a time during those years, averaging three hours of sleep a night for one entire year of school. He cut lawns at Boston University, worked in clinics, and even worked as a subject in medical experiments. "Hell," he told Noble, "one time I swallowed the tubes they needed to collect stomach content samples. I bartered for extra money, telling 'em that unless they'd give me more money, I wouldn't take the drug they were testing."

"What would they do?" Noble asked.

"There wasn't much they could do at that point, except pay me," he said, laughing at the memory. "I worked for a clinic, driving around Roxbury at night drawing blood and collecting throat cultures. I'll never forget one time I walked into this apartment building and knocked on the door I was supposed to knock on. The door opened and there stood the biggest black guy I'd ever seen. There was a Muslim flag on the wall behind him and he just looked down at me and said, 'What do you want?' I said, 'I'm the doc from Children's Hospital' and he just lit up. 'Come on in,' he said, and that was that. I'll tell you, if you can draw blood from an eighteen-month-old black kid squirming on his own couch with his mother holding him, you can draw blood from a turnip. You know, I really treasured those jobs."

But all the jobs, and the studying, and his having married so young took their toll. By the time Hannan graduated seventh in his class from Boston University Medical School (he was the third BU student in twenty-five years to be accepted for a residency at Massachusetts General Hospital), his marriage was on the rocks.

"How did you finally settle on neonatology?" Noble asked.

"Well, I could see that if I went into office pediatrics, all I was gonna do was wipe runny noses. Anything interesting and the kid would go to some sort of specialist. When I was finishing up my stint in the Public Health Service I found out they had an opening for a Fellow at Boston Lying-In, so I decided to give it a try. I'd liked working in the nursery during my residency, and Christie [whom he'd met during his residency and began dating and married after his divorce] was very supportive of the idea. And besides," he added, "neonatology is the last bastion of the generalist, which was what I wanted to be."

"Generalist, what the hell are you talking about? How much more specialized can we get?" asked Noble, puzzled by Hannan's remark.

"Think about it for a minute. The only way we're specialized is in the size and age of our patients. Okay, we don't do surgery, but we can sure as hell do it on an emergency basis. We aren't tied to one organ system or another. We treat all the systems, and we know more about each of those little buggers' systems than most of the specialists we consult. We're involved in treating every problem and every area."

"Then why bother to get consults?"

"Well, first off, as soon as you start thinking, 'I'm the only one who's got the facts,' you mess up. We have to consult. We may know damn well the kid's got a duct. We may know damn well nothing can be done for a kid with nothing in his skull. But it's always good to get another view, another perspective, a different approach. You know what he's going to say, although he may surprise you sometime, but you bring him in anyway to hear what he says. And also to make sure you've covered all the bases."

"But isn't that wasting everybody's time and money?"

"Not really. First off, you're showing compassion for the parents. You can tell them, 'We tried everything we could, and we consulted with Dr. Knowitall, the eminent specialist, and we're afraid there's no more that anyone could do.' You've freed them of that nagging doubt that maybe there was just one more person who could do something, or something a specialist would have found that you had missed.

"Also," Hannan continued, "if you ever find yourself on the wrong end of a witness stand and some turkey's asking you, 'How do you know you did everything you could for little Ralphie, doctor?' you've got that consult in the record. Your ass is covered, or as covered as it can ever be. And, obviously, you need the consult because if a kid needs specialty care, that care's going to be provided by a specialist. Remember baby Henry, the kid with the intestinal problem?"

"Yeah, the blockage."

"Right. Well, we thought we knew what the problem was, and it turned out we were right. But the kid needed a surgeon, and, even if we'd been wrong, we needed someone else's opinion on that one. Anyway, like I've told you before, you don't get sued when the kid dies. Maybe the OB gets sued, but that's not your problem. You get sued when you give the parents a defective kid."

"You've never been sued when a baby died?"

"Never. Hell, I told you about the kid who got too much salt. We told the parents we had killed the kid. Nothing. But give them a kid who weighed six hundred grams at birth and is perfectly normal other than being blind, or a kid who's lost part of a foot because he needed IVs for so long but is normal in all other respects, and look out! Sometimes the administrators say, 'If you're going to get sued, drop the bill.' But that's bullshit. Either you did right or you did wrong. And you don't settle things by adjusting bills. Well, enough of this. Here we are."

Noble looked up just as Hannan pulled the car into a little parking area beside the road. To their left lay a set of railroad tracks, below which ran the empty remains of the old C&O canal. And further down the slope, below the canal, ran the Potomac River. Hannan organized their gear and handed Noble a short graphite fly rod to use with his garbage-bag waders. Hannan, on the other hand, was fully equipped, complete with chest-high waders, fishing vest, net, fly collection, knife, and other paraphernalia. The two crossed the road and the railroad tracks and then slid down the coal-covered embankment to the canal below. After they clambered down the stone canal wall, Hannan warned Noble to watch out for copperheads in these rocks. "They like to sun themselves there."

"Great!" shouted Noble, jumping back. "You warn me *after* I climb down the rocks."

"Didn't want to scare you by telling you before," said Hannan, laughing. "Come on, let's get you set up." He led Noble out onto a series of huge boulders jutting out into the Potomac, which consisted of a series of rapids at this point. Hannan tied a leader and fly on Noble's line while the Fellow pulled his green trash bags over his sneakers and wrapped them around his thighs with strapping tape. "Christ Almighty! You look like the lower half of the Incredible Hulk," Hannan told him.

"I didn't want to invest in a pair of boots for my first trip. I might drown and never get to use them again. And this arrangement should keep me dry enough anyway."

"Okay. Now look. I'm going to work my way down the river a bit. You ought to stay around here and work these riffles." Hannan pointed out smooth areas, chutes, leading into the different patches of rapids. "Cast across here," he said, "for the head of the chute, and then strip line in toward you." He demonstrated a few casts and then watched as the neophyte clumsily imitated what he had been shown. "No. Look at me. Hold the rod in your right hand; let out some line, that's it. Now play it like a whip. Right, back and forth, back and forth. Now, let it go! That's more like it." And with that bit of encouragement he moved down the river, leaving Noble to work the rocks.

After about twenty-five minutes of catching nothing but leaves and logs, Noble began to pay more attention to the scenery than to the fishing. He lay the rod down and sat on the rocks, looking across the river to the cliffs on the opposite bank. The cliffs and slopes on both shores looked, with their fall foliage, as though someone had stood at the top and spilled cans of bright yellow, orange, red, brown, umber, and green paint down the slopes. The far cliff was bathed in shadow, but Noble could still see the colors. Golden eagles, vultures, and hawks circled lazily, climbing hundreds of feet on the thermal currents rising from the river beneath the cliff. Noble was lost in his own thoughts on the sun-warmed rocks when a sharp whistle brought him to with a jerk. He looked around quickly for the source of the sound and saw Hannan, about a quarter of a mile downstream, pointing upstream past Noble. The Fellow looked in that direction and saw a giant osprey, a fish hawk, shooting toward him down the river about 12 feet off the water, searching for its dinner. Then, just as the bird passed in front of Noble, it dropped straight down, talons extended, and emerged carrying the biggest fish Noble had ever seen outside of a market. He looked back down the river and saw that Hannan had already moved farther down. "I don't like to just sit in one place," Hannan had told Noble on their drive to the river. "I try a hole, see what's there, and then move on. There's no point in just sitting somewhere where there's no fish."

"Just," thought Noble, as he watched the receding figure of his boss, "as there's no point in practicing medicine where there isn't a constant challenge. Hell, he doesn't fish to get away from the pressure; he does it to get away from the people and their demands. He's as serious about this as he is about the nursery. If it isn't hard to do, it isn't worth doing. And if you don't do it perfectly, don't do it. It's a hell of a way to live if you can really pull it off. But you sure don't make many friends that way. You may earn respect, but you don't get many votes for being lovable," thought Noble. But then, what was it Hannan had told him several times?

"Sometimes I get accused of not paying enough attention to the social amenities, and that can hurt. But I'm not in this business to win popularity contests. If I'm trying to save some kid's life and I have to run over my best friend to do it, I will."

Chapter Eight

A sharp knock on the office door brought Hannan back from his daydream about trout. "Come in!"

"Jim. Got a second?" asked John Noble, sticking his head into Hannan's office.

"Ya. Come on in. What's up? Anything new with Alvarez?"

"No, but we've got a new problem. One of the nurses down-stairs in C Nursery thought she heard a murmur in one of the term babies down there and tried to get a hold of the private pediatrician . . ."

"And she couldn't get him, right?" asked Hannan, guessing at the rest of a too-familiar tale.

"Right. She called his office but they said he'd already gone home for the day and . . ."

"Well, hell, it's after 5 P.M. on Christmas Eve. We can't ex-pect a doc to hang around his office taking care of kids."

"Well, anyway, the nurse called the service and they said

they'd call the man but nothing happened. So she called two more times and he finally called back. Said he can't come in and wants the baby transferred up here. I went down and listened. The kid's a little sweaty, a tad dark. I think it's at least a VSD [ventricular septal defect], and maybe something worse. Should we get a consult and set up an ECG?"

"Shit! What else can we do. I have to call Fred Morris over at Children's anyway to check on that baby we sent over last week. I think they were going to operate today," Hannan told Noble, "so I might as well take care of all this at once. By the way, who was the private pediatrician? Al Johnson?"

"Right."

"Jesus H. Christ! One of these days I swear I'm gonna strangle that bastard!" Hannan spat out, jerking forward in his chair and slamming both palms down on the desk top. "He and I have had so many go-rounds I can't even count them anymore. I've got a file this thick"—he held his hands about three inches apart—"documenting our problems with him."

"He does this a lot?"

"That ain't the half of it. He's always dumping babies up here because he doesn't want to haul his ass up from the dinner table, or in from the golf course, or up out of bed. And some poor parent, or insurance company, to be more precise, is always getting stuck with a day of ICN care at $450 a day because some baby's got a rash on his butt."

"Can't you do something about it?" asked Noble.

"Well, in the first place, it's not just Al who does it. In the second place, I've done a lot about it. When I first came here the private pediatricians were getting us to do all their work and they were doing the billing for it."

"How so?" asked Noble.

"Well, some baby would be discharged along with his mother on a Sunday morning. The private doc wouldn't want to come in to do the discharge exam, so one of the Fellows would be called down to the nursery to do it. But then the private pediatrician would bill the mother for the exam. It's a hallowed tradition in medicine, the old when-I-was-in-med-school-and-in-ternship-I-was-a-slave-so-now-that-I'm-out-in-practice-I'm-en-titled-to-have-slaves-of-my-own syndrome."

"How did you stop it?"

"I just made it clear that whatever we did, we were going to bill for. They weren't pleased about that, but the administrator backed me and there wasn't a whole hell of a lot they could do about it. The thing that's always driven Al Johnson crazy is that anytime he sends a baby to us or asks for a consult, I make a note of my findings in the chart."

"What's wrong with that?" asked Noble, whose political naiveté always amazed Hannan.

"For one thing, then he can't bill for what we did. For another, I'll write notes that make it perfectly obvious the baby didn't belong on our service, like, 'This otherwise-healthy baby was referred to the ICN for examination of a rash on its butt when the private pediatrician was unavailable to come in.' I discovered at one point that he was ripping my notes out of the chart, so I've always been careful to write them on the same page as his notes, and, where I can, I write them above his notes. Hell, I don't mind helping out a private doc when he's stuck if he's somebody who's willing to help us out with a little teaching, or whatever. But we sure as hell aren't here to cover ass for some guy who wants to sit at home and charge for our work. Anyway, enough of that. I've got to call our mothers and I still have to touch base with Fred Morris, who I'm sure is going to be leaving for his home and hearth soon. So, anything else?"

"Nope. I'll head on back across the hall and see how many IVs have pulled out since I came over here. It seems all I have to do is walk out of there for five minutes and half the babies need their IVs restarted."

"Goes with the territory," Hannan told him, reaching for his cardex.

"Merry Christmas, if I don't see you later," Noble said as he walked out of the office.

"Same to you, John," said Hannan distractedly, his mind already occupied with the daily task of calling every mother whom he hadn't already seen in the nursery during the day. He started today with a call to Charlotte Fontain, whom he had seen earlier. But he had finally succeeded in making arrangements for Becky's transfer to St. Francis, and he wanted to make sure that Charlotte Fontain understood those arrangements. He dialed the number of the office at the Department of the Interior where Charlotte Fontain worked as a secretary. One ring. Two rings. Three . . .

"Hello, Charlotte? This is Dr. Hannan over at Metropolitan. Fine. No, nothing's happened with Becky. I just wanted to let you know we've finally arranged to have her transferred over to St. Francis. I'm afraid it's going to be tomorrow afternoon. I know it's Christmas but we've been waiting so long to get it done I didn't want to risk fouling things up by postponing it a day or two. The surgery? No, they won't operate until Monday.

"They're planning to come over here to pick her up at 2 P.M. tomorrow. Sure, you know you can come any time. In fact, if you want to you can ride over with her in the ambulance. No, it's no trouble at all. I'll be here myself. No, Dr. Javed will probably be going over with her, but if you have any questions he can't answer, don't hesitate to ask me. Right. You're sure you don't have any more questions about what we're doing? Okay then. As soon as we know any more, we'll talk to you, but I don't expect to know anything until Monday. Thank you, and Merry Christmas to you, too."

Hannan hung up, glanced at the cardex, and began dialing the next number. "Yes," he thought, "poor Charlotte's going to have a really Merry Christmas." The phone rang once, twice, three times . . . ten rings. And yet another failure to reach baby Smith's mother. "Probably out making her Christmas connection," Hannan thought bitterly. He dialed another number and listened to the rings.

"Hello. Mrs. Morrison? This is Dr. Hannan. Fine, thanks, and you? I'm just checking in to say no news, which is good news.

Everything seems to be going well. He's still doing well on room air, and the cut look's like it's healing nicely. No, I know we talked about the possibility of infection, but, as I explained, that was the worst possibility. No, quite frankly I'm surprised by how well it's healing. No problems at all. Are we going to see you today? Well, I'll probably see you tomorrow then. Afraid so. Somehow the boss always seems to get stuck with the duty. Right. See you then."

Hannan then dialed a series of six numbers, flipping through medical journals as he waited in vain for someone to respond to the ringing, and then moving on to the next number. The rhythm was broken by Rita Andrews who stuck her head around the corner of the doorway to announce, "I'm leaving now, Dr. Hannan. Should I turn the answering machine on?"

"What?" asked Hannan, looking up suddenly from *Pediatrics.* "Don't want to give me a full day anymore, huh, Rita?" joked Hannan, glancing at his watch. "Sure, you go ahead; leave me to spend my holiday evening here."

"Well, if you need me to stay—" Rita began.

"No," Hannan interrupted. "I was just kidding. You go ahead. And do turn the machine on. I'll turn on my bellboy. Have a Merry Christmas!"

"Same to you," called Rita, who was already halfway into the hallway.

"Jesus," thought Hannan, "I don't think I'm going to get hold of anyone today. Probably all out, doing last-minute Christmas shopping." And just as he completed the thought, a woman answered the phone. Caught off base, Hannan had to glance quickly at the cardex to recall whom he was calling. "Mrs. Adams? This is Dr. Hannan, over at Metropolitan. . . . I hope so, but I'll probably have to stay late this evening. You all ready for the holiday? Good. Listen, I was just calling to let you know everything's fine and Cato appears to be doing well. Yes, his weight's coming up. No, I'm afraid I didn't put it in my notes, but I know he's gaining well. Yes, his breathing's fine. No, no new problems at all. I can't guarantee anything, but I think he might be ready to go home shortly after New Year's. But as we've told you, there really is no knowing with these little babies. We missed you today," said Hannan, adjusting the phone between his neck and shoulder and leaning forward toward his desk. "You'll be in to-morrow? Good. Maybe we'll have a chance to talk. Good. Merry Christmas to you and Mr. Adams, too." He hung up the phone and flipped through the cardex. "Hell, I'm not going to get any more today," he thought. "Might as well try to get hold of Fred Morris."

It was almost 5:30 by the time Morris was able to respond to Hannan's call. The neonatologist was writing letters when the phone began ringing and was just about to let the answering machine take over when he remembered he had placed a call to Morris twenty minutes earlier. The machine had, in fact, begun to play back when Hannan picked up the receiver. "You have reached the Metropolitan Lying-In Hospital Division of Neo-natology. Nobody is in the—"

"Hello," Hannan cut in. "Hang on a minute while I switch this thing off. There. This is Dr. Hannan."

"Jim? Fred Morris, returning your call."

"Hi, Fred. Thanks for getting back to me so soon. I didn't know if I was going to get you before you headed home for the holiday, or if you were going to be tied up in the OR."

"No, I finished up down there a few hours ago, but I was up in the ICU checking on my patients. What can I do for you?"

"I hate to tell you," Hannan began, "but we've got a baby who just came up from the regular nursery. Yeah, term. One of the nurses picked up a murmur and he's looking a bit cyanotic. It could just be a VSD, but one of the Fellows thinks it's more than that. I was wondering how things look over there for Monday. I assume you're not doing anything over the weekend. . . . Right. No, I think it can wait. But I'd sure as hell like to get a consult as soon as possible to decide just how long we can wait. I wonder if you could mention it to Jack Cooper over in cardiology. I'd have called him myself, but I wanted to check with you anyway to find out how things are looking for baby Holt."

Hannan listened as Morris told him that the baby transferred to Children's Hospital National Medical Center the preceding day was, as Hannan had suspected, in need of open-heart surgery. The infant had a VSD, a ventricular septal defect, or a hole between the two lower chambers of the heart, as well as a malfunctioning mitral valve. "Well, that explains what we were hearing, anyway," Hannan said. "When are you scheduling her for? Tuesday? Good. Let us know how things turn out. By the way, when is baby Spencer scheduled for? Weren't you going to do her some time soon? Today? Terrific. The parents must be relieved anyway. I'm glad to hear it went well. Everybody over here really liked them. Well, I'll let you run. Let me know as soon as you've gotten things lined up for this new baby. I don't know the name myself. I'll check and leave it with your service. Okay. Merry Christmas to you, too."

After he hung up, Hannan left his office to go check on baby Alvarez; across town, in his larger, brightly lit modern office, Fred Morris prepared to leave for home. "Boy," he thought as he straightened his already immaculate desk, "Megan Spencer's surgery did go smoothly. Which is lucky, considering we had that reporter there." Morris had agreed to allow Bernard Daniels, a medical writer for *The Washington Post*, into the operating room to watch Megan's surgery. Daniels was working on a story about the recent advances in open-heart surgery on infants and young children, and Morris, who had worked with Daniels on a previous story, had decided to take a chance again. Members of the OR team hadn't been so sure. In fact, when the subject had been broached in a staff meeting two weeks earlier, most team members had been opposed to having a reporter present. Megan, they reminded Morris, was one sick little girl. She had already undergone cardiac surgery at the age of one month and now, at three months, was about to undergo an open-heart procedure. She still weighed only 9 pounds, 6 ounces, little more than her birth weight. She was having difficulty breathing and was obviously in a great deal of discomfort. There was a good chance as Jack Brennan, Morris's chief resident, reminded his boss, that Megan might die on the table. And how would that look in *The Washington Post?* But Morris had decided to take a chance on Daniels and the story. And thus at 7:45 A.M. on Christmas Eve, Morris was standing outside the men's dressing room attached to the hospital's surgical suite, waiting for Daniels to get into a scrub suit, mask, cap, and booties.

"Have we got a few minutes to go over some background?" Daniels asked, emerging from the dressing room. Morris glanced at his watch.

"Sure. Why don't we go into the lounge?" Like everything else in the gleaming, ultramodern hospital, the physicians' lounge was spacious, well lit, and decorated with bright colors and comfortable, modern furniture. The contrast with Metropolitan Lying-In, Daniels thought as he sat down, was appalling.

"How common is the procedure you're going to be doing today?" the reporter asked Morris.

"We've done ninety-nine patients with isolated VSDs—kids in whom this was the only problem—since 1974. This will be the one hundredth. Of those, we've done thirty-one patients less than a year old. The numbers have increased each year. There were eight deaths, which is about the national average."

"What, exactly, does having a VSD mean?" Daniels asked, taking notes as Morris spoke.

"Normally the two systems in the heart are separate," Morris began, "with the red blood on the left side of the heart under high pressure and the blue blood on the right side under low pressure. Realistically, the heart is two hearts, each with two chambers—one, on the right side, that pumps the blue blood to the lungs, and the other, on the left side, that pumps the red oxygenated blood to the body. Now what happens as a result of the VSD is that the red blood comes back from the lungs to the heart, and instead of all of it going out to the body, a major portion of it seeps through the hole, back to the right side of the heart and to the lungs again. For Megan, for every one quantity of blood that gets out to the body, three go back to the lungs."

"Does that mean she isn't getting enough oxygen?"

"No," explained Morris, "but it means her heart has to work four times harder than normal to supply oxygen to the organs. It's a tremendous metabolic insult."

"If just a few years ago you were waiting until these kids were three, four, or five months old to operate, what was happening to their systems?" Daniels asked.

"They used to suffer a lot more permanent damage, including pulmonary hypertension. We used to use a technique called pulmonary artery banding, which didn't require the use of a pump. We just went in and put a constricting band on the pulmonary artery. What that did was restrict the flow of blood to the lungs and protect the lungs from damage. But it didn't deal with the high pressure in the heart, so the heart wasn't totally protected. Then we had to go back in later, remove the band, and repair the hole in the heart. Now the approach is a one-stage technique, to take care of everything in one sitting while the kiddie is still in infancy."

"Are there any medical treatments you can use?"

"Yes. But they're just stop-gap methods. We can use digitalis to treat the heart failure and diuretics to get rid of some of the fluid that builds up as a result of the heart failure. And there's also something new we've gotten in the last year called 'after load reduction.' What that does is lower the resistance of the body's blood vessels, making it easier for the blood to go out through the aorta rather than back through the hole and into the lungs. It acts on the smooth muscles of the blood vessel walls. You take a little piece of medicated tape, like Scotch tape but with medicine in it, and slap it on the baby's back. It's graded according to how much medication you need. She was getting a quarter-inch of tape four times a day."

"How long can you delay surgery?"

"We used to wait until the babies were three or four months old, as long as they maintained reasonable growth patterns. But as we found we could do it safely, we've been operating on younger and younger children. It's been this way with a lot of things in medicine, and in life for that matter: When you're forced into doing something with a little higher risk and realize that you can do it, it changes your outlook and approach to things. The next time around, you realize that you can do it earlier and earlier."

"So you started by doing the operation on babies you were convinced would die without it, and then realized it was safe to operate on such young children?"

"That's right," Morris told the reporter. He glanced at his watch again. "We'd better get in there now and see how they're doing."

At 8:11 A.M., Megan Spencer lay on her back on the operating table in the center of Operating Room 2. Her head was turned to her right, her eyes taped shut. Her pale white skin contrasted sharply with the halo of bright red hair rising from her head. Suction tubes arched across her face, from her mouth to her ear and off the table. The loudest sound in the room was that of her heart, amplified and broadcast by a loudspeaker as it tripped along at 162 beats a minute. A black tube the size of a garden hose lay across her body like a black snake, attached to the smaller clear plastic tube that connected Megan to the anesthesia equipment. After checking to see that the anesthesiology team and Jack Brennan, Morris's senior resident, had everything under control, Morris turned to go scrub. "Jack, could you get towels and bolster up the cooling pad?" he asked Brennan and then, to heart/lung machine technician Bob Jamison, "Bob, could you get it from your side? I want it arched up so the cooling and heating are against her skin." The pad would be used to help bring down Megan's body temperature for the surgery, slowing her metabolism and decreasing the amount of oxygen needed by the various organs.

"What's most likely to go wrong?" Daniels asked Morris over the roar of water rushing into the scrub sink.

"Usually irregular heart rhythms," said Morris, scrubbing his arms to the elbow. "Bleeding that we can't control is rarely a problem at this age. Then there's the possibility that the heart just won't start up again on its own after surgery because of its extremely stressed preoperative state. Plus it has the additional insult of being on the pump, and having anesthesia and incisions and patches and sutures. Though the heart is fixed at the end of the procedure, there's no guarantee it will work properly. The hole will be closed, but the price to be paid is a significant insult to the pump's efficiency. Whether that insult lasts for an hour, six hours, sixteen hours or six days is a variable. That's where the Intensive Care Unit plays such an important role. But this kiddie has the kind of lesion which would lead me to expect her to be awake and responsive to her environment tomorrow morning. We'll keep her on the respirator a day or two, just so we can keep her at rest, control her breathing and oxygen input. You ready?" asked Morris. He had pulled a blue cover gown over his green scrub suit. A fiber optic light sat on his head like a miner's lamp; the metal-wrapped cable carrying the light-transmitting fiberglass cord hung down his back like a tail. When he stepped up to the operating table, the end of the cable would be attached to a box containing a high-intensity light source. The light would then travel along the cable to the lamp on the front of his forehead. "Let's go," said Morris, who, holding his still-dripping hands in front of his chest, shoved the door to the OR open with his hip.

At 9:02, his wet hands clasped before him, Fred Morris stepped toward the table on which Megan Spencer lay, her back arched by the towels Morris had ordered placed there. The surgeon held out his hands while Inez Garcia, the circulating nurse, helped him into his filmy latex surgical gloves. The massive light over the table bathed Megan's chest and groin area in a pool of white light, which quickly turned a brownish red as Morris and

Brennan painted her entire body, from groin to neck, with Betadine, an antiseptic wash. The solution ran over the sides of her rib cage and disappeared onto her back, briefly creating tiny abstract paintings on the canvas of her skin. A plastic Steridrape with a sticky backing was smoothed across her chest and abdomen, and the two men then draped her entire tiny body in pale green surgical towels, covering her legs and lower body and her head and face and leaving only her chest, covered with the translucent Steridrape, exposed. By 9:11 Morris was checking the valves in the tubing that would carry Megan's blood from her body to the heart/lung machine and back to her body.

Finished with the preliminaries, Morris glanced at the clock. It read 9:13. "Are we ready to start?" It was a statement, not a question. With one deft move Morris used a scalpel to draw a 4-inch line down the center of Megan's chest. At first the razor-knife appeared to leave no mark, but then a thin red line appeared along the path of the silver blade. Wisps of smoke rose into the air and wove their way through the light beam bathing the baby's chest. The smoke, and the stench that accompanied it, were caused by the cauterizing tool with which Morris burned shut the dozens of blood vessles he had cut with that first incision. It took just five minutes of cut, burn, cut, burn, cut, and burn to open Megan's chest to the point where stainless-steel spreaders, which looked a bit like a modernistic picture frame, could be placed in the chest to hold the two halves of the rib cage apart and allow access to the heart.

As Morris sliced through the pericardium, the protective envelope around the heart, Bob Jamison and his team were preparing the "pump" that would sustain Megan's life while her heart was being repaired. The so-called heart/lung machine really consisted of three separate pump circuits, as well as an automobile tape deck that Jamison had designed into the custom-built unit. "What are you doing at this point?" Daniels asked, after introducing himself to Jamison.

"Right now we're just priming the pump," said the perfusionist. "First of all, we've done some calculations. We've figured out the child's circulating blood volume so we know the volume of our circuit. We've tried to work out some numbers so when the child's on bypass, and on our circuit, the hematocrit [the percentage of solid elements in the blood] will be thirty. Then we take the blood and we buffer it. We've brought the pH up to a normal level and we've added calcium. Now we're taking this blood from the blood bank that we're priming with and we're recirculating it to bring it up to a temperature that will approach the patient's temperature. They're cooling her down right now. She's—" he paused as he glanced at one of the instruments—"she's ninety-six now and the cooling blanket's sixty-five. When we hook her into the pump, the blood temperature of the pump will be set to meet her temperature so it won't be a shock to her system."

"Look at this," Morris called to the reporter. "Here's a dramatic demonstration of the whole process. This," he said as Daniels approached the table, taking care not to step into the sterile area, "is a huge pulmonary artery. You'll have to take our word for it," he said with a laugh, "but it's huge. It's probably three times larger than normal. This is the aorta here. Normally, in kids the pulmonary artery is half again as big as the aorta. But here it's four times bigger. This is very, very impressive."

Megan's overworked heart lay beating rapidly in her chest, exposed for all to see. "We will be able to use standard perfusion," Morris called to the pump team. "We'll use a four-three and a four-four. We're going to have to use a ten in the aorta because it's really small."

"No way we can use a twelve?" asked Rich Barnum, Jamison's assistant.

"No way. I don't know how we're even going to use the ten," replied Morris, who was inspecting the lines as they were being sewn in place in the superior and inferior vena cava, where the blood will be drawn to the pump before it can return to the heart from the body, and into the aorta, where the pump will return the oxygenated blood for circulation throughout the system.

"These are fine," Morris announced, inspecting his associates' work. "We're waiting for the partial occlusion clamp and the purse string sutures." Almost as soon as he received what he asked for, Morris asked for more sutures. "Let's check the pressures," he said and used a probe to make a direct measurement of the pressure in the right and left ventricles and main pulmonary artery. The pressure on the right side of the heart should be approximately half that on the left, but the numbers called off by anesthesiologist William Goldman told a different story:

"Right ventricle is sixty-two, sixty-three," said Goldman. "LV is seventy-seven. Main pulmonary artery is sixty-three."

"We're ready with the blood," Jamison announced from his post by the pump.

"Pump and suckers are set," Morris responded.

"That's enough blood," said Jamison, as the first flow began into the pump.

"Give it a hand turn," called Morris, and the pump crew responded by checking each of the individual pump units.

"We're just about ready to go on the pump," Jamison explained to Daniels. "We check redundantly to make sure that all the pump equipment is right before we go on. We check again and again. Some teams don't do that. But the point is, if you went on the pump and then had some sort of problem, the pump equipment does not become a factor in your thinking, when you're trying to figure out what the problem is. You've already checked it out, so you can eliminate it as a source of the problem."

"Okay," said Morris. "We're in the aorta and we're bubble-free. The clamp is off. Okay. We're on the pump and cool the body to twenty-eight [82.4 Fahrenheit]."

"You're on bypass," Jamison told Morris, as the blood began to leave Megan's system through the clear .15-inch line, through a junction into a quarter-inch line and into the pump, where it

would be cooled and returned to the body through similar lines.
"What we do now is stop the heart," explained Jamison, as the
reporter continued to take notes. "We use a solution called cardioplegia, which is high in potassium. It's pumped right into the
coronary arteries and shuts the heart down."
"What's the temperature?" asked Morris.
"Temperature is twenty [centigrade] and coming down rapidly," Rich Barnum told him. "Eighteen and still pumping to
you. Okay, 11 degrees [51.8 Fahrenheit]. Finished cooling."
"What we did," Jamison said, continuing his explanation of
the process, "is put a very small needle right at the coronary
arteries and then put a clamp across the aorta right behind the
coronaries. As we pump the cardioplegia in, it must go into
the coronary arteries; it can't go anywhere else. It goes only to
the myocardium, and the high potassium shuts down the electrical system in the heart, turns it right off. The solution is also
designed to provide all the substances the heart needs to maintain viability, and it's cool, so it reduces the need for oxygen."
As Morris worked within the confines of the tiny chest, the
loudest sound in the cavernous operating room was the incessant
slurping noise of the "suckers" drawing blood out of the chest
cavity and into the pump, where it would rejoin the circulating
blood and return to the body. The sound was not unlike that of a
child trying to get the last drops of a milk shake up through a
straw. But Morris was oblivious to the noise and quickly found
that he could get to the pea-sized hole in Megan's heart without
actually cutting the heart muscle itself—a discovery that greatly
improved the long-term outlook for the child.
After making a small incision in the baby's pulmonary artery,
Morris worked his way down through the valve, exposing what
turned out to be an elliptical hole between the two lower chambers of the heart. Because of the shape of the hole, the surgeon
was able to simply draw its edges together with a patch, sewing
it closed and using minute Teflon bolsters to plug leaks. Less
than twenty minutes after the pump went on, the repair had

been completed. Morris then used clear saline solution to check the repair for leaks. "Look at that. Not a drop is coming out," he announced. "Fantastic! Fully rewarm," he told the pump team, who then began to reverse the process and warm Megan's blood. It was 10:32, exactly thirty minutes since the pump had taken over the work of Megan's heart and lungs, circulating and oxygenating the blood.

"Coming off the aorta," said Morris. "Clamp's off the aorta," he announced.

"Are we making urine?" asked Jack Brennan, wondering whether Megan's kidney's were functioning properly.

"I think so," Morris told him. He glanced down at the clear plastic receptacle connected to the catheter in Megan's urethra. "Yup. We're doing well," he told Brennan after noting the yellow fluid collecting in the bottom of the container.

"Temperature's 30 and coming up," announced the pump crew.

"What we're doing now is inserting a pressure monitor directly into the left side of the heart," Morris told Daniels, who stood by the head of the table, wedged in between the anesthesia equipment and the monitors and watching the surgeon, "and we'll take it out tomorrow morning. It helps us to know the filling pressures in the business side of the heart. Temperature?" he asked the pump technician.

"It's 31."

"This went too smoothly," Morris joked. He was a quiet, competent but totally unassuming man, outwardly lacking the traditional surgeon's ego. But the operation had, in fact, gone so quickly and easily that Morris was forced to bide his time, waiting for the blood to rewarm.

"Let me have an inside sucker on the aortic needle vents," he called.

"You've got it."

"How long have we been on pump? We're ready whenever you are," said Morris.

"We've been on forty-six minutes," Jamison told him.

"Please. Please. Please. Please. Please," muttered Morris, trying to will the blood to warm faster. "What's the temperature at the head?" he asked Goldman.

"Its 32," the anesthesiologist told him. "Now it's 32.7."

It was 10:46 A.M. "We'll come off pump at 34" [93.2° Fahrenheit], announced Morris. The minutes ticked by as Morris moistened the heart with what looked like a basting bulb filled with saline solution.

"Okay. You've got 34," Jamison told Morris eight minutes later.

"Let's go off the pump," Morris told the team.

"You're off," Jamison told the group, and Megan Spencer's heart was on its own once again.

"Pressure's 70 at 7.6," said Goldman, checking his instruments. "90 at 7."

"What's her temp?" asked Morris.

"It's 34.7," Goldman told him.

"Okay, here's where we get our test marks," said the surgeon, waiting for the complete pressure readings.

"Reading 58 right ventricle," Jamison announced. "Pulmonary artery 57. Left ventricle 105."

"That's it, then," said Morris, who watched as Jamison wrote the numbers down on a large recording board at the end of the room, next to the preoperative readings of 63 in the right ventricle, 77 in the left, and 63 in the pulmonary artery. There was now a clearly marked difference between the pressures on the right side and on the left side of the heart.

"I'm going to see my patients," said cardiologist Arthur Tate, Megan's physician, who had been observing the surgery. "I'll check in with her parents and let them know everything's gone well."

At 11:21, as Morris and his team went about the business of closing the incisions, the speaker was once again turned on, filling the room with the flub-dub sound of Megan's heart. This time, however, it was beating at only 122 beats a minute, rather than the 162 beats per minute of a few short hours ago. It took the surgeon and his chief resident thirty-three minutes to sew the incision closed, using wire to draw the two halves of the sternum together, and then finer and finer sutures for each succeeding layer of tissue. Morris's needle work on the layer just below the skin of Megan's chest looked like fine embroidery, bringing the skin so close together that there was, for a second time, only a fine red line down the center of her chest. There were no stitches placed in the skin itself. Instead, at 11:53, Morris lay fifteen short strips of surgical tape across the incision, drawing the skin closed.

Goldman began the business of undraping Megan, removing the surgical sheeting from her head. "Hello, baby," he said to the still-anesthetized child. A bed was wheeled in to carry her up to the hospital's pediatric Intensive Care Unit. On it lay the pink, yellow, and blue wool blanket Megan had been clutching when she had been put to sleep four and a half hours earlier. The child was moved to the bed by an attendant, and as Goldman adjusted the oxygen supply and Megan's endotracheal tube, Morris looked down at the naked baby lying spreadeagled on the bed. "Little frog," he murmured, smiling as he gently stroked her foot.

Chapter Nine

It was close to six o'clock before Jim Hannan realized he had forgotten to call Christie to let her know he wouldn't be home for dinner. Ordinarily he and his wife, a nurse-researcher at both Metropolitan and St. Francis, might have ridden home together. But Christie had finished her work in Metropolitan's follow-up clinic by 3:30 and had gone home to finish preparing the house for the holiday.

Hannan dialed the number by memory and reflex, not even glancing at the dial. "Hi! I'm afraid I'm going to be late tonight," he told Christie when she answered. "We've got a terrible problem over here, a new baby that came up with multiple anomalies, and we're trying to decide . . ." He paused and listened. "No, no, that baby hasn't even been delivered yet. This is another kid and he's on a respirator and passing meconium through his penis and has no anus and has a cardiac defect and chondrodystrophy and big, doughy, masses which are probably ureters. We had to put him on a respirator on one hundred percent oxygen and it's the first baby and the parents are all upset. About three hours ago. An elective cesarean. Dick Benjamin," he told her, answering her questions. "Hell, we've already had Bob Albert and Arnie Greenberg come over and give us their educated guesses. Just what you'd expect. Bob said he could correct what he could see, but that depends on whether the kid had kidneys and on what Arnie Greenberg says about the heart. Who? Arnie? What do you think? He said he thought it was worth taking the kid over to St. Francis for a cath and a workup. Of course he also said the odds were the baby would die on the way or on the table. I know. Well, I laid it all out for the parents and they opted to wait until morning and see how things look then. Ya. They're upset, but at the same time they're amazingly together. Especially the mother. She's really an incredible lady. They're not particularly sophisticated, but they know damn well what's going on and what they want to do about it. What? Oh, ya.

"No, go ahead and feed the kids and don't save me dinner. I'll grab something here," said Hannan, fiddling with one of his yellow pencils. "Yes, I know what night it is, but there's just no way I can get away early. I know it happened last year, too. That's the way the game is played. Give the girls a kiss. No, wait, put them on the phone.

"Hi, Cathy! Sorry I can't come home to help you hang your stocking and read *Winnie The Pooh* with you, but I have to stay here. Got a little baby that's sick. It's got a lot of problems. It's very, very sick. Your child has a little sickness?" he asked, smiling at the thought of his youngest daughter's "sick" doll. "Well, I'm sure it will get better. Did you have fun today? You did? Good! Let me talk to Maggie, okay? I love you, and I'll kiss you when I get home.

"Hi, Mag! How was your day? You did? Did you tell Mom? I'm going to have to teach you a little more jujitsu so when that happens people will learn not to fool with you. Okay! I love you, too! I wish I could but I really can't. Okay. Put Mom on.

"I'm glad I talked to them," he told Christie, "because I probably won't get home before they're in bed. By the way, how did follow-up go today? Four? Christ, that's about as good as you've ever done. Sure I remember. That bad? Well, what can you do? That's right. Well, I better get back over and check on the Alvarez kid. That's the baby. I'll see you later on. You too." Hannan hung up and dragged himself out of his chair. He wanted to go back to the nursery to give baby Alvarez another examination. He also had to work out the evening's coverage with John Noble and let him know when to call Hannan in, if need be.

As Christie Hannan stood in her kitchen at home, working on the chestnut stuffing for the Christmas goose Jim had shot earlier in the fall, her thoughts turned to the difficulties of trying to run the unit's follow-up clinic on any sort of scheduled basis. Mothers would promise to come in and then not show up, or show up on the wrong day. They'd start in the program and then drop out. Rich Sherrill, one of the unit's three fully trained neonatologists and director of the follow-up program, had explained the problem succinctly to the medical students this afternoon, Christie thought.

"There are many reasons for lack of attendance," began Sherrill, sitting behind the desk crammed into the suite of three tiny rooms that the hospital's employee health service lent to the follow-up clinic for an hour and a half a week. "They include lack of transportation, single-parent families where the single parent works or has other parenting obligations, and just other priorities, especially kids who have multiple problems. It's more important for them to get primary care, or therapy, than to come here. I think the only way we could improve attendance," he told the students and Ravi Javed, who was also working in the follow-up clinic this afternoon, "would be to buy a van and hire a driver with liability insurance and actually go out and pick the babies up. There are some programs that do that.

"The worst part of the poor attendance is what it does to our data," continued Sherrill. "Statistically what we don't know, of course, is whether the segment that doesn't show up is better or worse than the median. Our attendance rate has been about sixty percent. I don't think it will get any better unless we combine this with primary pediatric care, and we're not about to go into that business," said Sherrill of the program strictly designed to measure and monitor the mental, motor, and neurological development of low-birthweight babies who passed through the nursery.

"How do these kids stack up, compared to term babies?" asked medical student Martin Wells.

"The really low birthweight kids will, on the average, lag behind babies who were born at full term," explained Sherrill, "but if you correct for prematurity, they will do about the same as or better than babies born at full term. Actually, what the—" The *beep! beep! beep! beep!* of the hospital's page system interrupted. "*Dr. Sherrill,* six-seven-six-five, *Dr. Sherrill,* six-seven-six-five." Sherrill picked up the receiver of the telephone on the desk and dialed extension 6765. "This is Dr. Sherrill. Was someone trying to reach me? Uh-huh. Yes. No. Tell him to wait until I get up there. About three-thirty. All right," he concluded, hanging up the phone.

"As I was saying," Sherrill began, resuming his lecture, "what the literature suggests is that, growth-wise, if the babies are born the appropriate size for their gestational age and get reasonable nutrition in the immediate post-birth period, they will come up into the normal growth range. Head circumference will usually be the first to catch up, which is of course what we'd hope for— because of the brain—and then length. Overall weight will be the last. The overall weight is probably the most misleading indicator of physical development. As you might expect, head and overall length are far more important indicators.

"Usually you'll see accelerated velocity of growth during the first year," Sherrill continued. "In terms of the motor development, again the literature suggests that somewhere between thirteen and fifteen percent of the very low birthweight babies, probably below fifteen hundred grams, have significant handicaps. If there's going to be a significant motor handicap, you'll usually see it by one year of age. It's a little harder to predict what a child's whole performance is going to be. There's some data to suggest that if you look at his mental performance around two years of age, you'll have an indicator, but it's really difficult. One of the things you've got to look for is delays in language development. This may indicate a problem with sensory input, such as hearing, or it may indicate mental retardation. It's one of the things you start to pick up around two, three years old.

"I think the key times to look for abnormality are, say, at one year, in terms of motor handicap; then at two years to see what mental performance is, and then when the child gets to school. You may not be aware of kids' having significant mental problems, or language difficulties, until they get to school. Right here we're just following them for two years for motor, mental and neurological development. But to really do a thorough, comprehensive, follow-up assessment you need to do more things. We don't pretend to have a comprehensive program," Sherrill told the medical students, who were leaning against the walls of the cramped office for want of chairs.

It used to be thought that saving tiny prematures, weighing 1,500 grams or less, would increase the number of mentally and physically disabled children and adults in the population. In older studies, researchers in this country and in Scotland found that up to 60 percent of very low birthweight babies who survived had substantial physical and mental deficits at five years of age. And before 1960, 7 to 12 percent of surviving premature babies had the most common form of cerebral palsy. However, in the decade between 1960 and 1970, that number declined to less than 4 percent. And recent surveys of the medical literature show that by the beginning of the past decade, between 80 and 90 percent of the babies born at the best of the nation's perinatal centers did not suffer from any serious mental or physical handicaps. Even more recent studies, however, including a major program in Canada, have found that up to 48 percent of the low-birthweight survivors enter school with a major learning disability or other handicap. The verdict on long-term survival is clearly not in yet, and, in fact, it may never be. For there are no studies, including the excellent Canadian work, that match low-birthweight premature babies with their term counterparts, eliminating such variables as IQ of the mother and father, home environment, educational level of the parents, their attitude toward education and achievement, and a host of other environmental and hereditary factors that can affect a child's performance in school and in life.

The team at Metropolitan has studied "forty kids at one year of age," Sherrill said, "and less than ten percent had serious handicaps. We don't correct for gestational age here, which some groups do. We just look at the test performance. A lot of prematures come in and by one year they're within the normal range."

"What do you mean when you say 'major handicaps'? " asked Saul Goodman.

"Major disorders means loss of one or more limbs, gross seizure disorders, or hydrocephalus. Those are major handicaps. You have to remember," cautioned Sherrill, "there are a certain number of kids with gross defects who are going to die during the first year. In that low-birthweight group, mortality during the first year is significantly increased. The reason for that is sudden infant death, which is significantly higher in that group. Respiratory death is higher in the low-birthweight group, especially in kids who had respiratory problems and were on the respirator. And a third cause of death is gross defects: If a kid had an intracranial hemorrhage at birth and developed hydrocephalus, he's got a much better chance of dying. The single most morbid neonatal diagnosis is intracranial hemorrhage."

"What about putting a CAT scanner in the unit?" asked Martin Wells.

"That's only going to diagnose them, not cure them," Sherrill answered.

As Sherrill was talking to the students, Christie Hannan was administering the Bayley motor development exam to Charlene Arnold, who had spent the first seventy-five days of her life in the Metropolitan ICN. "What are you feeding her?" asked Christie as Roberta Arnold struggled to get her tiny daughter out of an equally tiny snow suit.

"Formula," said Roberta, a quiet, reserved woman.

"With iron?" Christie asked.

"Without; and a vitamin daily."

"Good. Do you know how much she weighs?"

"No. I think about six pounds," said the baby's mother with an embarrassed laugh.

"When's the last time you took her to the pediatrician?" Christie asked.

"She hasn't been yet."

"Do you know who you'll be taking her to for private care?"

"Probably Dr. Jenkins," said Roberta, freeing her four-and-one-half-month-old daughter from the grip of the pink and yellow garment.

"Good. What we'll do today is go ahead and test her. We'll do a motor test and a mental test and a neurological test. We'll then send the results to Dr. Jenkins' office. If we feel she needs any special tests or help, we'll tell you what we feel and then make recommendations to Dr. Jenkins. All right?" Christie then turned her attention to the baby, who was staring at her intently with enormous deep brown eyes that seemed to take up half her face. "Hi! Hi! You're such a big girl now! Yes, you are!" She paused in her cooing to notice that Charlene's mother still had a coat on.

"Wouldn't you be more comfortable without that?" Christie asked.

"I guess I would," said the woman, laughing again as she shrugged her way out of the slightly worn, bright red winter coat. Just as Christie was about to begin testing the baby's motor development, the two medical students and Ravi Javed walked into the examining room and crammed themselves into the little bit of space not taken up with an examining couch, small table, sink, and two chairs.

"You'll be amazed how many talents she has that we can test for," Christie said as she placed Charlene on her side and watched as the baby kicked out her legs and flopped onto her back. She then repeated the performance, placing the baby on her left side. That accomplished, Christie propped the infant into a sitting position and watched which way she fell, noting whether the child tried to put out her hands to protect herself. "Does she like being on her tummy?" Christie asked Roberta Arnold as she placed the cooing infant on her stomach on the examining couch. "What we're looking for now is both crawling and holding up her head." The baby raised her head ever so slightly from the white paper covering the green vinyl surface of the examining couch, but she made no effort to crawl. Christie then shook a rattle in front of the baby, but the infant made no attempt to reach for it or follow it. "I'd like you to hold her in your lap now, if you would," said Christie, handing the baby to its mother.

"Charlene. Look at this, Charlene. Charlene. Take this," said Christie, waving a bright red plastic ring back and forth within the baby's reach. Charlene began to reach for it tentatively and finally, encouraged by Christie's prompting, grabbed the ring. "Very good, Charlene!" Christie said warmly, encouraging the baby. "Now let's try these." She placed three yellow blocks, each the size of a sugar cube, on the table in front of the baby. Again, with much encouragement, Charlene tentatively reached forward and then grasped first one, and then another of the blocks. "Do you notice she's reaching for things at home?" Christie Hannan asked the baby's mother.

"Sometimes she does," the woman told her.

"Good. That's very good. All right, I'll have to take her from you again for a minute," said Christie, reaching for the Pamper-and-undershirt-clad child. "That's a girl," she said, lifting the baby from her mother's lap. She then lay the baby on its back on the examining couch and pulled her up by the arms, watching to see how stiffly Charlene would hold her back and neck. "Very good!" Christie told the child and, more importantly, her mother, as Charlene maintained some rigidity in the line of her neck and back. "Okay. Why don't you go ahead and feed her now, and Dr. Doyle will be in in a moment to do the mental test." Christie, the two medical students, and Javed then extricated themselves from the cramped, stuffy room and stepped back out into the equally crowded office area. Within half a minute, however, Dr. Mary Beth Doyle, a developmental psychologist from St. Francis, entered the room. She was trailed by the same students and Fellow, who once again had to find places to wedge themselves.

Many of the tests administered by Doyle appeared to be the same as those already used by Christie Hannan. She shook a rattle and noted whether the baby followed the rattle with her eyes as it was moved from side to side in front of her face. She did. The same test was then repeated with a bell, with similar results.

"Has she started smiling yet?" Doyle asked Roberta Arnold.

"Yes," the woman told her.

"Do you have to work a lot to get her to smile, or has she started to do it on her own?"

"Oh, she smiles some on her own."

"Will she 'talk' back to you when you talk to her?"

"Oh, yes. It doesn't sound like much, but . . ."

"No, we don't look for a whole lot of meaning," the psychologist explained. "Would you say she has a lot of different sounds, or just one sound?"

"She has different sounds," said Roberta, whose baby was beginning to let loose a barrage of squeals and grunts as she became frustrated with the colored blocks.

"That's what I'm talking about," said Doyle. "What are you getting upset about?" she asked Charlene. Doyle then took the block and placed it on a foot-square sheet of colored plastic that she held in various positions at and below Charlene's eye level. The psychologist banged the block on the sheet, attempting to attract the baby's attention. "Sometimes at this age they'll look at things across eye level but not really be able to look down yet," she explained to the baby's mother. "She's so friendly," Doyle said, and then she turned her attention back to the child, noting that "this isn't your favorite thing, is it?" She substituted a green Flair pen for the block and sheet, waving it back and forth in front of the child's face. Charlene reached several times for the pen, seemingly unable to grasp it with her stubby fingers. Finally, however, she grabbed the object and immediately drew it toward her mouth. "You almost got that in your mouth," Doyle told the child. "That's another item on the test! Did you say to Mrs. Hannan that you've seen her trying to reach, or not?"

"Yes, I have," Charlene's mother told the psychologist.

"Have you ever seen her feeling her fingers?"

"Every now and then."

"Does she stare at them and move them?" Doyle wanted to know.

"Sometimes," the woman told her.

By the time Doyle had finished with the mental exam and Richard Sherrill came in to administer the neurological portion of the test, Charlene Arnold was becoming frustrated and irritable. She was fidgeting in her mother's lap and alternately whimpering and bawling.

"Hi, Mrs. Arnold, how are you doing?"

"Okay."

"Good. What we're going to do now is test her reflexes. I remember you well," Sherrill told the baby, who couldn't have cared less. "You do look a little different though." As he took the baby through the various phases of the test, checking her deep tendon reflexes and her head control, suspending her to see whether her feet reflexively began a walking motion, Sherrill talked to the medical students and Javed, explaining to them, rather than to Roberta Arnold, what he was testing and how he was doing it. When he finished, he and the rest of the group left Roberta Arnold and her baby in the examining room and gathered in the office area to discuss their findings.

"Okay, I think we can start to summarize now. I think in terms of recommendations, the usual thing I would recommend would be range of motion exercises [which improve the baby's motion through its joints]," Sherrill told the students. "Mary Beth, do you have any specific recommendations? Christie? No? Okay. Oh, Mr. Arnold?" said Sherrill, glancing up at a large black man who had just entered the office and who looked slightly confused. "Your wife is in the examining room. You can go in and we'll join you in just a minute to go over the test results with the two of you."

"How long you gonna be?"

"We'll be ready in about five minutes," said Sherrill.

"Five minutes? Then I won't go put another quarter in the parking meter," said Delbert Arnold.

"Actually, you might go put it in," Sherrill warned him. "Your wife is still going to have to dress Charlene and get everything pulled together." As Arnold left the room to go feed the parking meter, Sherrill and the team returned to the examining room to explain the test results to Roberta Arnold.

"We just want to review these results with you," Sherrill told her as she struggled to get Charlene back into her snow suit. "First, you have to remember these tests are all geared to full-term babies. Charlene was eleven weeks early, so you have to take that into consideration. Now, on the mental exam she scored a little over three months, so that's quite good. She's a little over four months old, but she was born two months early. On the motor examination she scores at two-and-one-half months, which is also quite good. There didn't appear to be any specific weaknesses or problems. On the neurological exam, which I did, her muscle tone is slightly increased, and by that we mean she had a little stiffness in the legs and arms, not a lot: in fact it's less than I see in a lot of babies who come back at this age. The only specific recommendation I would have for this would be to do what we call range of motion exercises. You take each joint, the ankle, the knee, the elbow, the shoulder, and the wrist, and move them back and forth and side to side. Do the exercises when she's relaxed, like after giving her a bath. Do you have any questions about anything we did?"

"No," the baby's mother said quietly.

"I would think she probably needs to encourage her to look up a little," Christie Hannan added. "Place Charlene on her tummy and place things out in front of her so she'll have to look up."

"That will help her neck," said Mary Beth Doyle. "At this age that's the main sort of challenge. There are two things: One is to start using her hands, which she's doing; the other is to hold her head up. She'll be doing that more naturally, but you can help her. On the tests that I did she's really doing beautifully."

"I think you're both doing a great job," said Sherrill, taking note of Delbert Arnold, who had quietly slipped into the room and was now standing behind his wife. "I'll send our report to your private pediatrician. Do you have any questions, Mr. Arnold?"

"Things such as her navel aren't in your area, right?" asked Charlene's father, who was apparently worried by the fact that her navel protruded slightly.

"No. You'll have to check with your pediatrician about that," said Sherrill. "We're just checking developmental things."

"Babies don't wear belly bands anymore?" asked Arnold.

"No. Okay, if that's it then, we hope to see her again. Mrs. Hannan can give you another appointment."

"This first visit was really just to give us something to compare with to see how she's doing later," explained Mary Beth Doyle. "There really aren't many things she's supposed to be doing yet. Do you have any questions or worries that you want to bring up about her development?"

"Yes," answered Charlene's mother. "Do you feel like you're seeing her make much progress?"

"It's too early to talk about progress," said Sherrill, "but from what we saw today, we can say she appears to be doing very well. Anything else? All right then. Have a Merry Christmas and we'll see you in a few months." With that Sherrill and the students left with Javed, leaving Christie Hannan to make an appointment for the baby's next visit.

"Navel. Did you hear that?" Mary Beth Doyle asked Javed. "I don't know what it is, but all the fathers seem to spend their time worrying about their daughters' belly buttons. Jesus!"

"What have we got next?" Javed asked Sherrill.

"Mrs. Isherwood is waiting in the other examining room. Mrs. Hannan's done the motor, so why don't you do the neurological?"

"Right. Who's got baby Jones?"

"Mrs. Hannan's going to do the motor on her now, and then Mary Beth will take the mental and I'll get the neurological," said Sherrill.

Javed, followed by the two students, walked into Examining Room 2, where a well-dressed woman sat playing with her chubby, grinning, eight-month-old son. "Long-lost friend! You're happy to see me?" Javed asked the beaming baby. "Come on, let's go! Say 'hello' to them," Javed told the drooling child, whom he picked up and placed on the examining couch. "Okay, let's sit down and see what you can do. Boy, are you heavy. Let's make you sit like that so I can hold you from behind," he said, placing the baby in a sitting position. "Where do you expect a baby to fall?" he asked the students.

"Forward?" Martin Wells volunteered hesitantly.

"Yes, that's right," Javed told him. "Usually the forward protective reflexes are the first to develop, then the lateral, and then the posterior." He tipped the baby forward, and little Kinte put out his hands to stop himself from toppling. He did the same thing when pushed to the right, and then the left. "He has some protective reflexes and some balance," said Javed of the laughing, still-drooling baby. "What you have in the first three months are usually just the primitive reflexes, the autonomic reflexes are developing during this period. Then during the three-to-six-month period he'll get control over the hips, and from nine to twelve months he'll gain control over the lower extremities." A ringing telephone in the examining room interrupted him.

"Hello. Yes, he's here," said Martin Wolf, who had answered the phone. "Yes. I'll tell him." He hung up. "It was the blood bank," he told Javed. "They wanted to tell you the blood is ready for that exchange transfusion."

"Good. I'll get up there as soon as we finish." He picked up the baby and held him as the child moved his legs in a walking motion. When he was held still, Kinte's chubby legs supported his weight. He cooed and shouted, seeking attention for his accomplishment. "He can bear his weight on his lower extremities okay," said Javed, "now let's see what he likes. Down on your back," he said, lowering the baby down. "Now, go for it, take it!" He waved a pen in front of the infant, who waved his hands at it and reached for it, quickly succeeding in grasping it. Javed took the pen back and waved it again. "Come on! You can get it! Go for it! Observe the type of grasp he has," the Fellow told the students. "Come on! Don't just smile, grab it! There! You see, he still has entirely a radial grasp. See, the usual development of grasp is palmar grasp first, then it goes to more or less ulnar, then it progresses to midpalmar, and then to radial, okay? Then finally you get a pincer grasp, which is usually around this time. Now, let's see if he has transference. There, you see, he's trying to reach with his mouth." The baby, lying on his back in his blue rubber pants and Superman T-shirt, began to cry in frustration. "There, there," said Javed, giving the baby the pen. "I was about to say that's the time they usually start to scream."

After placing the baby, who had stopped crying almost immediately, in various position, Javed observed for the students, "He has good head control; he can look up, look sideways. He's beginning to use his upper torso. Next he'll start to use his hips, and that's called crawling. Then he'll use his upper thighs and hamstrings and he'll lift himself off the ground and start scooting. Okay, I'd like you to hold him in your lap," Javed told Cynthia Isherwood. "Usually, with so much voluntary movement, it's difficult to obtain reflexes in a baby like this. But if the tone has increased, you can usually tell." Javed used his small rubber hammer in an attempt to elicit a full set of reflex responses. "He has some increased tone in the lower extremities," he told the mother and students, "but the upper extremities are quite okay." He worked with the baby's neck and then asked one of the students, "If I have two babies, one on its front and one on its back, and both of them are three months, which of them will be able to turn over?"

"The one on its front," Saul Goodman told him.

"Okay. Why?"

"Because they can turn over just using the upper torso."

"That's right," said Javed, who, observing Kinte's movements, told the baby's mother, "I think he's going to be crawling quite soon." After a brief conversation with Cynthia Isherwood about her son's developing interest in speaking, Javed placed the baby back in her lap. "You'd better hold him for this last part," he said, "because he's not going to like it very much." He then took a cloth tape measure and quickly checked Kinte's head circumference and length. He was not quick enough, however, to keep the baby from bawling. "Okay. Okay! You can go home now.

Take it easy," he told the infant, who did, in fact, relax and begin to smile again. "We'll be right back," he told the child's mother, and the Fellow and two students retired to the outer office.

Javed sat at the desk in the outer office scoring the baby on the exam sheet. "Mrs. Hannan saw some problems with the motor," Sherrill told him.

"When he's reaching for objects, he doesn't really reach," Christie told the group, "he has a sweeping motion. But he did do it once."

"I saw some increased tension in the lower extremities," said Javed, "particularly in the ankles."

"I think what we're more worried about," said Sherrill, "is that he has a tendency to extend all the time, to push his legs straight out."

"But he can roll and he can flex," said Christie.

As Javed continued filling in the sheet for the little boy who had entered the nursery weighing just over two pounds and didn't leave the ICN for forty-four days, Christie and Mary Beth Doyle were having a brief discussion about baby Jones, a little girl who was also eight months old. Unlike the two little boys, who seemed to be doing relatively well for their gestation age, Leticia Jones, the two women noted, was a sad case. Her grasp was poor, her reach was practically nonexistent, her muscle tone and control were poor, and she did very poorly on the mental test. They were comparing their test results when Sherrill began to sum up the findings on Kinte Isherwood.

"Let's see. The baby four months ago was at three point two months in the mental and is now six point five, so he's progressed three months in that time. He's progressed three months in the motor during that time, which is less than we'd expect. Neurologically, this is interesting, because last time we didn't note any problems with tone or range of motion. That's my concern now."

"I think she's encouraging the standing up," said Mary Beth Doyle, who, like Sherrill and Javed, believed that Cynthia Isherwood was working with her son, trying to get him to stand up, which was causing him to extend his legs so much.

"I know," said Sherrill, "and I think we better discourage it."

Once again the entire group trooped into the examining room.

"Okay," began Sherrill. "We're all set. Let me review the results: First, if you remember from the last time, our tests are based on full-term babies, and Kinte was, of course, born two months early. On his mental exam this time he scored six-and-one-half months, and on his motor exam he also scored six-and-one-half months, so his motor and mental are on the same level, and he was born a couple of months early, so they're both within the range of reasonable development. But there are a couple of things we're concerned about. Number one, we feel he needs to develop the ability to reach for objects—small balls, blocks, things like that."

"Reach?" asked Cynthia Isherwood, clearly puzzled.

"Right, reaching out. Okay?"

"Okay."

"That's very important during the first year because the baby is developing the ability to use the thumb and forefinger to pick things up. That's something you want to work on in the next two months. Also, have you had his eyes checked?"

"His pediatrician's seen him, but I don't think he's checked that. Dr. Franklin saw him when he was here."

"But he hasn't been checked since leaving the nursery?" asked Sherrill.

"No."

"Well, he should be seen by somebody. It doesn't have to be Dr. Franklin if his office isn't convenient to you. But it should be checked.

"The third thing," continued the neonatologist, "and I may have mentioned this in the last visit, is that we want you to do range of motion exercises with him. It's particularly important in the lower extremities. And the fourth thing is, we don't want you to encourage him to stand up. I think the most important thing is for him to be sitting and crawling. Standing will come later. I notice he has a tendency to extend his legs and try to stand. But other things are much more important now. Okay," said Sherrill, slapping both palms down on the tops of his thighs, "do you have any questions about anything he's doing or anything we've done or told you?"

"He's a little backward because he's a premie, but he's doing all right?" asked the baby's mother.

"Yes. Overall, his development is within the range of what we'd expect for his prematurity. I've told you the things we're concerned about."

"All right."

"We'll send a full report to your pediatrician, and he can use it to add to his impressions and observations. We'd like to see Kinte again at twelve months. By the way," concluded Sherrill, "did you take him up to the nursery?"

"Not yet."

"Well, if you have the time, the nurses would really appreciate it. They only see sick babies and tiny babies, so they enjoy seeing the babies when they're strong and healthy. You weren't at the Christmas party last week, were you?" asked Sherrill, refering to the ICN's annual Christmas party for survivors and their parents. More than fifty children, ranging in age from four months to five years, had attended the recent gathering.

"We were both working," explained Cynthia Isherwood.

"That's okay. But I'm sure the nurses would really appreciate it if you could stop by for a few minutes."

"We will," said the child's mother, as she began dressing Kinte in his pants and sweater.

"Have a Merry Christmas, and say hello for us to your husband," said Sherrill, as he rose to leave the room.

"I will, Dr. Sherrill, and Merry Christmas to you, too."

Chapter Ten

It was 8:30 P.M. before Jim Hannan could finally lock his office door and head home to enjoy the few remaining hours of Christmas Eve. A lengthy reexamination of baby boy Alvarez had proved no more conclusive than the earlier examinations and consultations. The infant's condition hadn't worsened any in the past few hours, but neither had it improved. Hannan went over the case in detail with John Noble, who was the Fellow on call for the night. If there was any change in the infant's condition, Hannan was to be called. Because no decisions had yet been reached, if the baby arrested or took a turn for the worse, Noble was told to proceed with the same life-saving procedures he would use in any other case. Decisions not to resuscitate, or to make a less-than-wholehearted effort, were not ones that Hannan ever delegated. Nor were they decisions he wrote in the record, or anywhere else for that matter. It was one thing, he believed, to reach such a decision in concert with a sick baby's parents and then act on that decision. It was another thing entirely to leave a written record of that act, a record that would be read and misinterpreted by anyone who happened to obtain a copy of the chart.

The dry, powdery snow squeaked beneath the rubber soles of his L. L. Bean boots as Hannan walked across the parking lot to his car. A sixth sense told him that he would be called back to the hospital before dawn. He wasn't sure what would necessitate his returning, although a change in baby boy Alvarez's condition was the most likely possibility, but he knew with a certainty born of fifteen years' experience that he would, indeed, be back.

Just as the atmosphere in the nursery had become more tense when Hannan entered it for rounds eleven hours earlier, so it relaxed when he left for the day. Freed of the constraint of having the boss looking over their shoulder, the nurses chatted and joked more among themselves. The atmosphere may also have been lightened by the fact that the evening shift saw the heaviest volume of visitors, as parents unable to take time off from work came to spend what time they could with their sick babies.

Martha McNeil, who sat in a white rocker in the middle room feeding her daughter, Beth, was a fixture on both the evening and day shifts. On most days she would spend as many as eight or nine hours in the nursery, coming in the early afternoon and leaving with her husband about 9 or 10 P.M. She had been in a good mood the past week, for now, after a forty-day stay, it looked like Beth would be going home in time for New Year's. But as Laura Crowley, a senior nurse on the shift, finished feeding baby Breslin, who was in the next Isolette, she noticed that Martha McNeil's shoulders were shaking ever so slightly, as though she were crying and trying to hold in the sobs. Laura tapped Sally Mitchell on the shoulder, and Sally, who had was just making notations on a chart, took Susie Breslin from Laura.

"Martha? Are you all right?" Laura asked the woman.

"What? Oh, sure. I'm fine," she lied, wiping a tear and a

strand of long black hair from her eye with the same motion. "Really. I'm okay," she told Laura, who was looking at her in disbelief.

"Listen. That bottle looks like it's empty and it's time for my break. Why don't we go have a cup of coffee together in the nurses' lounge. Come on."

"Thanks. I think I'd like that," said Martha, rising from the chair. She carefully laid Beth, who was already asleep, in the Isolette, and quietly closed it. She stood looking down at her daughter, once again lost in thought, until Laura lightly placed a hand on her arm.

"She'll be all right," she said softly, guiding the woman from the room.

The nurses' lounge, two doors down the hall from the ICN, was decorated for Christmas with a 3-foot-high artificial tree and a string of colored lights across one corner of the closetlike room. The effect was depressing, rather than cheering, and accentuated the institutional nature of the small, stark lounge area. Laura poured cups of strong black coffee from the stainless-steel urn on the counter and handed on to Martha. "Try this," she told the woman. "It may make you sick, but then you won't think about being depressed."

Martha took a sip and immediately made a face. "Gosh! This really *is* awful!" she said, setting the cup aside. "I'm sorry I was being so silly in there," she said sheepishly. "I try not to lose control, but . . ."

"But you wouldn't be human if you didn't on occassion," said Laura, finishing the sentence for her. "Don't think you're the first mother we've seen cry," she continued, "and don't be embarrassed by it. It's the mothers who don't cry that we worry about."

"I know. It's just that I feel so silly, behaving like that with her coming home next week. I guess I just got to thinking about Christmas and everything Beth's been through and everything we went through with Sam . . ."

"Sam? He's your little boy, isn't he? What happened to him?"

"You don't know? I thought everybody up there did. This isn't my first stint in the ICN, you know. Sam was there for forty-seven days and for at least a month of that time we didn't really think he was going to make it."

"Oh, my God!" said the young nurse, her hand rising involuntarily to her mouth. "How have you held up this long?"

"It really hasn't been that difficult. It was a shock, all right, when I delivered prematurely again. But it's been a lot easier for us this time. We've known what was happening. We're familiar with the equipment and the procedures, and with a lot of the staff members. And Beth hasn't really been all that sick. As you know, her hyaline membrane disease wasn't that bad. She had a patent ductus but it never presented any real problems. She was on the respirator, but only for a couple of days, and then she was on oxygen for a while. It's just been an entirely different experience from what we went through with Sam."

"You had a rough time with him?" asked Laura.

"Awful. In the first place, I started out with a rocky pregnancy. I had some spotting at eight weeks and the doctor told me to stay home for a couple of weeks. He said it was not unusual, but he wanted me to stay in bed until it stopped."

"You were a public health nurse in Baltimore County, weren't you?"

"That's right. And I went back to work after the spotting stopped. But then, when I guess I was about three-and-a-half months pregnant, I started having some really heavy bleeding, so he put me to bed again and this time I stayed in bed almost two months. Then I was up again and then I was back in bed. Then, when I was about twenty-eight weeks pregnant, I started to hemorrhage one afternoon. I started bleeding around five and called the doctor around six. He told us to come right in to the hospital and it was about seven by the time we got here. I had stopped bleeding by that time, so I felt like the perfect fool."

"Wait a minute. You live out in Ellicott City, don't you—up

near Baltimore? Then whatever possessed you to come to Metropolitan?" asked the nurse.

"I know that seems silly, but I've been using the same OB-GYN since I was a teenager and lived in Virginia. We'd been married for almost nine years before I got pregnant with Sam, so I really hadn't needed an obstetrican before then. I guess I was just comfortable with my doctor so I stuck with him. It did make for a long drive to the hospital though, didn't it?"

"I'll say. What happened when you got here? Did you deliver right away?"

"No," she replied, now able to laugh about that chaotic night twenty months earlier. "My doctor decided to keep me overnight for observation, and together he and I concluded that perhaps there was a source of bleeding that could be controlled when I was semi-upright. So he kept me in the hospital and told me to sit in bed. That helped, believe it or not. I was in the hospital a week and had very little bleeding. We even talked about my coming home. But at just about that time I had more bleeding and simultaneously went into labor."

"Did they deliver or try to delay labor?"

"They tried to stop the labor with alcohol and some other things, but it just proceeded," Martha told her.

"What did your OB tell you about the baby's chances? I know the things we hear some of them tell mothers are really awful," said Laura.

"He told me Metropolitan had very good results, but with the baby being as small as he was, and as early, I think he said it had maybe a forty to fifty percent chance. At the time, they had taken me off the regular OB floor and put me up here. My parents were making daily trips to see me and they'd walk down here to the ICN and look through the windows at the babies. Then they'd come back and report to me, 'Oh, those babies aren't *that* small. They don't look that bad.' They were really very encouraging."

"What did you think was going to happen?" the nurse asked,

taking a chance that it would be best for Martha to talk out her fears and pent-up emotions of the past twenty months.

"I guess I was primarily worried about retardation," Martha told her. "I was personally convinced the baby's nutrition wasn't what it should have been, because of the bleeding. My OB tried to encourage me, telling me his wife had similar problems and their baby had grown up to be a normal, healthy young man."

"Did anyone from the ICN come down and talk to you beforehand—tell you what we were going to be doing and what you could expect?"

"No, and that would have been nice. That's the only thing you people could possibly have done to help that you didn't. Otherwise, everyone was just so terrific."

"How long did the alcohol drip hold off labor?" Laura asked.

"Not very. Of course, when it first started I denied the fact I was in labor and thought I was just having back pains . . ."

"That's very common," the nurse told her. "If you've been counting weeks, waiting to get to that due date, you just can't get used to the fact that everything's happening so early."

"I know, but I'm a nurse, for gosh sake!" responded Martha.

"You're also a woman," said Laura. "The same thing has happened to people who work in this unit."

"That's reassuring, because I was so convinced I was just having back pain from having sat up in bed all week. But by one A.M. there was no question what was happening. I was really devastated. I thought, 'This just can't be happening this way. This is the end, we've gone through all this bleeding, and spending time in bed, and our baby's going to be born dead or not be able to survive.' I thought that, in spite of everything we'd done, we were going to lose him. But both Herb and I have a real faith that God was in control of every detail of our lives, and I think that was the thing that gave us the greatest amount of strength. Also, we had many, many friends praying for us that night, and, I don't know, somehow there was a peace underlying everything that night. We were very, very concerned, obviously. I can't say we weren't. But we really had a peace to get us through."

"Was Herb there for the delivery?"

"He was out in the waiting area because it was too late for him to come in by the time he got down here."

"How did the delivery go?"

"The worst part was that when Sam was born there was some question about his sex. Nobody told me whether he was a boy or a girl. Nothing was said."

"That must have been awful," exclaimed Laura, involuntarily reaching across the small table to touch Martha's arm.

"It was certainly strange. The delivery room was absolutely silent when he was born because he didn't cry. I was just waiting for him to make any noise at all, but there wasn't any for what seemed an eternity. Then, finally, I heard a series of little gasps. After he'd been taken away, and I hadn't seen him at all, I asked the obstetrician whether the baby was a boy or a girl. He said, 'I think it's a girl, but when babies are born their genitals are sometimes quite swollen and it's difficult to tell.' So there were some concerns, of course. Later a nurse came and clipped a bracelet on my arm telling me it was a girl. It turned out Sam had hypospadias, and there was some confusion about sex."

"There's a baby up here now—baby Adams—who has hypospadias. You may have noticed the 'Do Not Circumcise' sign on the Isolette."

"You know, I noticed that with Sam but I never really asked what it was all about. I know that sounds incredible."

"No, there are a lot of things going on, and you aren't always going to focus on all of them. That sign's there to make sure a baby with hypospadias doesn't get circumcised. When they perform the surgery to correct the condition they need to use the foreskin to give them something to close that urethral opening running up the underside of the penis," explained Laura.

"Oh, that makes sense. Well, when Dr. Sherrill came to see me later that morning, he seemed confident that Sam was a boy. And Dr. Amis, who was a Fellow then—I guess that was before you came—was very reassuring, too. He said the child was definitely one sex or the other and they would determine which one it was and we shouldn't worry about it. But Herb had an unpleasant experience in connection with all of it. He was sitting down in the waiting area and heard the operator at the desk commenting on the phone to somebody, 'Well, I have to have the sex one way or the other! I've *got* to know.' And then she gave our name, so everybody in the area could hear it. It was just a harsh thing for him to have to go through."

"That's awful," said Laura. "They're usually pretty good about that kind of thing down there. But sometimes they just don't think about who may be overhearing them. So when did your husband finally get to see the baby?"

"He went up right away. He had to wait a bit while they got Sam ready. They had Sam set up on the warming table in the corner in the front room. Herb couldn't believe he was even seeing a baby. Sam had these deep, deep retractions, and every time he took a breath his sternum was practically at his back bone. It's hard for men to deal with newborn babies anyway, but to see your firstborn in that condition . . . He was quite shaken. But he came back to me and said he didn't know much about medicine, but he thought Sam was a boy, judging from what he'd seen. We started to get a little more confident after what Dr. Sherrill had said. And he suggested that we name the baby and try to get as close to him as possible during his stay in the nursery. It was quite an experience trying to decide whether to use a girl's name or a boy's name."

"How did you feel about what Dr. Sherrill told you about getting close to the baby? Were you concerned that you'd get close and then something would happen?"

"I don't think Herb or I ever had the experience of not wanting to get as involved and attached to the baby as possible. We weren't sure for a whole month whether he was going to make it. He was on the respirator, and then off and looking better, and then he took a turn for the worse and went back on. He had a good case of hyaline membrane and a patent ductus. He also had some other heart irregularities, and with all his lung problems he went into congestive heart failure. And on top of that he had hypothyroidism plus the hypospadias."

"What was your reaction when you saw him yourself for the first time?" asked Laura.

"If I'd been walking into the ICN to see somebody else's baby it would have been a lot different, but . . . I just felt like crying, falling apart. It was a shock. Having been a nurse, I knew there were just so many unknowns. And I was concerned about brain damage. To see him lying there! He weighed two pounds, fifteen ounces, so he was bigger than some of the babies, but he still looked so tiny and helpless. It was hard to imagine he would ever grow into a real child. I guess," she hesitated for a moment, "I guess our concerns were that if he did survive, what would his potential be as a child? It was very frightening. The staff was very, very reassuring, without being overly optimistic."

"Did you come down to see him every day the way you have with Beth? God, that must be hard," said Laura, who lived with a group of women in a rented townhouse two blocks from the hospital and considered anything more than five blocks a long commute.

"It was rough. It is rough," said Martha. "It's exactly a thirty-mile trip from our house to the hospital. I came down every day. A friend would usually drive me down in the mid-afternoon—that's what I do now—and then Herb would come down after work and we'd go back together in the evening. So between us we were covering ninety miles a day. With the forty-five days for Sam and the forty days so far for Beth, we've driven seven thousand six hundred and fifty miles!"

"Good God!"

"It really hasn't been that bad. Somehow you get used to it," said Martha.

"You know the thing I've noticed about you and Herb? You always seem so, I don't know, so serene together when you're here. So many parents get to blaming each other for what's happened and end up taking things out on each other or the baby.

I'm sure you've heard about the various studies, how the divorce and separation rate is so high in couples who have prematures, and that the incidence of child abuse is much higher among premature babies than among term babies," said the nurse.

"I've read some of that," responded Martha, "but we just haven't had any problems. There just hasn't been any blame. In some ways our days with Sam down here were days of real growing together. I know this sounds odd," she said, blushing slightly, "but it was a sweet time for us, in a way. We'd often stop at Giffords for an ice cream cone on the way home and sit there and talk and end up crying together. It's all been so different with Beth."

"How so?"

"To start with, I had a perfectly normal pregnancy—no complications. I just sort of assumed . . . well, after I had Sam I had a long talk with my obstetrician and he said he thought that what had happened with Sam was just a quirky thing, that I'd had the bleeding and the bleeding had acted as a stimulant to labor. He thought if I got pregnant again it would be a whole new ballgame. We'd be starting from zero again. But I guess in the back of my mind I was concerned that once I had a premature delivery, that would be the trend.

"But, I don't know. I hadn't really planned to get pregnant with Beth so soon after Sam, and I became pregnant quite easily. And everything was normal—right up to the day Beth was born. I did get a little anxious as I approached thirty-two weeks," Martha explained, "but the doctor assured me that everything would be fine and I'd go to term. When I went into labor I called him and he said it probably wasn't labor . . ."

"That's typical. You're in labor, you're experiencing it, and they tell you you're not in labor," said Laura, who was no fan of OB-GYNs as a group.

"I had what I thought was some show, but when I called him he said it was probably just a small blood vessel that had burst, and that I should stay in bed, just to be sure. I stayed in bed all day and waited for Herb to come home and take care of Sam.

Then, as the day progressed, I started to have some labor. I guess I began to feel it around four P.M. By six o'clock I was certain I was in full labor. Herb wasn't there at the time, but as soon as he came home—I think it was around six-thirty—we jumped in the car and drove down here. My obstetrician had told me to come in. He said they'd probably check me and keep me overnight. He obviously didn't believe I was in labor and it was happening again.

"I think my doctor was taken by surprise this time, but you never know with doctors," said Martha.

"You sure don't," Laura added.

"I kid him now that if I ever get pregnant again I'll plan for a premature delivery and hopefully be pleasantly surprised. *Anyway.* By the time we got to the hospital this time, I was fully dilated and Beth's feet were getting ready to be born first. The membranes hadn't ruptured yet, though, which was fortunate, because I guess if they had been ruptured she would have been born in the car, and that wouldn't have been too good for a breach birth."

"They sectioned her, didn't they?"

"Yes. But I was awake and she was in much better condition when she was born than Sam had been. I heard her cry right away. You know what's really funny? When we were here the last time I became quite friendly with Evie Roth, and when I was lying in the delivery room, she came running up to me and said 'Martha! What are you doing here!' She was on the Code Pink team that evening! Having gone through all this before, I knew somebody familiar would be in the delivery room, but I never dreamed it would be Evie."

"That's quite a coincidence" said Laura. "I haven't heard of that happening before. Of course we don't get that many repeaters like you. We have had several, though, since I've been here. What was it like for you, finding yourself up here with a second child? Did you have trouble separating the experiences in your mind?"

"At first it was difficult to accept because it was such a shock. I had no preparation, you know, that she was going to be a premature baby, except in my own mind. I was thinking she would be and hoping she wouldn't. So it wasn't the same as it was with Sam, where things had been going wrong all along. When I went into labor with Beth it was just like, 'Oh no! I can't believe this is happening to my life!' Our lives had just started to settle down. And to lie in that recovery room and think, 'The baby's already been born! Here we are starting all over again!' The first time hadn't been that long ago. Sam was only nineteen months old!" Her voice rose in frustration as all the months built up for her again. "To be finished with such a draining experience, finished forever, and then have it begin again. It was just unbelievable. A real shocker."

"But once you realized what was happening, as you mentioned a few minutes ago, wasn't it a little easier because you had been through it before?" Laura asked her.

"I think it was easier. I know that sounds silly, after I've just told you what a shock it was and all. And not that we wanted to go through it a second time. I certainly would have chosen to have Beth go full term. But I think the prior knowledge and experience helped. But, you know, it's almost impossible to compare the two experiences. With Sam we were on pins and needles for a month; we didn't know if he was going to survive. But Beth hasn't been like that. She's had many of the same treatments and procedures done, but they didn't concern us as much, like when they do PT, when they suction them, when they gavage them, when they do IVs, the constant heel sticks for blood gases. Sam's probably scarred for life, he had so many heel sticks."

"That's not exactly a major problem," laughed Laura. "Not many people are going to be looking closely at his heels. We've had at least one baby lose part of his foot because of abcess from the IVs they have to put there because there were no other veins left to use. So a few scars there aren't much. Has he been seen by a urologist yet for the hypospadias?"

"Oh, yes. We took him to Johns Hopkins. He had his first

surgery five months ago, and then he'll have the second, and final operation in about eighteen months. It's funny, in a way . . ."

"What is?"

"Our worrying about his sex, and the hypospadias. When we went to see the urologist we told him Sam's problem was so bad that we were worried it couldn't be corrected. Then he examined him and said, 'This isn't that bad. There won't be any problem achieving a total correction.' I guess that's what comes of seeing the problem all the time. To us it was something new and horrifying. To him it was just an everyday problem."

"Let me ask you something. We never see the bills on our end, obviously. If I can ask, what did it cost to have Sam with us for forty-nine days? I've always wondered about that. I mean, they tell us it can run over $100,000 if a baby's really sick, but . . ."

"Sam wasn't that bad. But it came to $17,000 for the hospital and another $4,000 for the physicians. So it was a total of $21,000. I guess Beth's will be a little less. Insurance paid the entire thing, but you know something? It would have been worth it even if it hadn't been paid. We knew we were well taken care of here, but we didn't know how well until Sam got pneumonia his second winter. That was a real nightmare."

"How so?" Laura asked.

"Well, he was admitted to Guthrie Memorial, outside Baltimore, with a pretty bad case of pneumonia. They put him in intensive care right away, which was fine, but then we discovered that we could only visit him twice a day for an hour each time! Here at Metropolitan, you were happy to have us in the ICN twenty-four hours a day, and we had been spending up to eight and nine hours at a time with this tiny newborn. But at Guthrie, when he was old enough to really know he was being separated from us, they wouldn't let us stay with him! It was frustrating and infuriating. I'm sorry to raise my voice again," said Martha, calming down a bit, "but every time I think about those people I just boil."

"I can certainly understand why," Laura told her.

"Then, then, our pediatrician decided he wasn't sure Sam was a boy! And without asking our permission he went ahead when Sam was in the hospital and ran another chromosome test. Do you believe it?!"

"I take it you switched pediatricians?"

"You better believe we did. The test, of course, showed he was a boy."

"My God, you've been through a lot," exclaimed Laura. "But at least you're going into the Christmas season with everything working out. Beth couldn't be doing better—I'll be surprised if they don't send her home in a week, unless something we don't expect happens. And Sam's coming along fine. So this is no time to mope. I know it sounds trite, but try to look on the bright side."

"No, it doesn't sound trite. I guess I was just feeling sorry for myself this evening—sitting here in the hospital on Christmas Eve with my second premie. Herb's at home with Sam, decorating the tree and wrapping the few things we haven't wrapped. And, you know, this is the first Christmas Eve he and I haven't spent together in the eleven years we've known each other. But you're right. Things could sure be worse. And the Lord has been pretty kind to us, when I stop to think about it. So I guess I better stop this and let you get back to work."

"Oh, gosh! I hadn't thought about the time. We've been in here almost an hour," said Laura, glancing at the watch safety-pinned to the waist of her green scrub dress. "It's just about ten o'clock."

The two women rose simultaneously, threw their used styrofoam cups in a metal trash can, and walked out the door. Laura fell a few steps behind Martha as the nurse reached back into the lounge to flick off the lights, a habit she had picked up in her group-living situation. Anything to hold down the utility bills, she thought.

Chapter Eleven

Although there were still more than half a dozen parents in the ICN at 10 P.M., the rooms and hallways of the rest of the hospital were devoid of visitors—at least they were supposed to be. But Stephanie Roberts had managed to bluff her way past the operator at the hospital's front desk and had simply walked to the elevator and pressed the "up" button. And so she stood, at that late hour, hesitating outside the door of Room 329, a massive bunch of hot-house daffodils clutched awkwardly to the chest of her down parka. She had been debating with herself during the drive in from her apartment in nearby Crystal City about whether she should be making the drive in the first place. It *was* late; she hadn't called Meg to say she was coming; and the baby had been born just eight hours earlier. But Meg and Andy had only been in the area three months and Stephanie was Meg's only friend who wasn't at least 500 miles away. When Andy had called earlier to tell her about the baby he had sounded a little hesitant—excited, to be sure, but Stephanie had gotten the feeling that something was wrong. And if there was something wrong with the baby, she was sure Meg wouldn't want visitors. "Well," she thought, "I've come this far, I might as well go all the way." And with that she reached out a mittened hand and rapped tentatively on the brown wooden door.

"Come in!" It was Andy's ever-cheerful voice.

Stephanie opened the door a foot and stuck her floral offering through, followed by her head. "Merry Christmas! Is the little mother receiving visitors?"

"Hi, Stephie! Come on in," responded Meg, who was propped up on two pillows in the hospital bed. She wore a lacy new bedjacket—a present from Andy—over her nightgown, and an IV board strapped to her left hand. The board was used to steady the needle and clear plastic tube leading from Meg's arm to the bag of clear fluid hanging above the head of the bed. "The flowers are beautiful! But you shouldn't have. They must have cost a fortune this time of year."

"Not really," replied Stephanie, hanging on to her flowers with one hand while she wriggled free of her coat with the other. "I got them from one of those street vendors for half-price just as he was closing up his stand for the night. But I didn't come here to talk about flowers! How are you? And even more important, how's the kid? A daughter, Andy tells me. I knew you'd come through with one for our side."

"Andy tells me she's beautiful," replied Meg.

"You haven't seen her yet?"

"No. I'm still pretty groggy from the epidural, and they've got me on Demerol for the pain. I saw her in the delivery room for a second, but . . ."

"Can't you go see her now? It's been eight hours; you must be dying to see your new daughter!"

"I think I'd rather wait till the morning, when I'm feeling a little better, and besides . . ."

"Oh my God!" thought Stephanie. "Here it comes."

". . . I really want to make sure she's doing all right before I go up."

"Up? Isn't she in the nursery down the hall here?"

"No. She's upstairs in the Intensive Care Nursery," said Meg, her reply trailing off into a whisper.

"Intensive Care?"

"It's just a precaution," Andy interjected. "She was born about three weeks early, and they said she was having a bit of respiratory distress." The way Andy said it, it sounded like nothing more than a mild cold. Stephanie was alarmed nonetheless.

"Oh, my God!" she exclaimed, immediately regretting her reaction.

"Oh, don't worry," Andy said, trying to calm Stephanie and his wife, whose eyes were welling up with tears. "It's just a precaution. Really!"

"Andy's been telling me that all afternoon and evening," Meg told her friend. "He talks as though respiratory distress was something every baby gets. Well, I know. It's not!

"They only let me see the baby for a second in the delivery room, so I knew something was wrong. But he's been calling everybody," she gestured toward Andy, who was looking sheepish, "and saying 'It's healthy, it's healthy,' and I keep saying they wouldn't have taken her away if she was. I've seen many deliveries and they always bring the baby up and show the mother, and my baby went by so fast I couldn't really see her. I just turned my head and they were walking out." Here she paused to wipe her eyes with a Kleenex from the box on the bedside stand.

"Uh, look. Would it be better if I left and came back later?" Stephanie asked, feeling incredibly awkward. She and Meg had been good friends from the moment they met in their apartment house laundry room a week after Meg and Andy had moved to the Washington area. But their friendship had been built on the superficialities of everyday life. And now, Stephanie realized, as she squirmed in her hospital-issue, straight-back chair, she really knew very little about Meg's background and her relationship with Andy.

But Meg didn't want Stephanie to leave. It helped, she thought, to have an outsider there with them. Somehow it made things easier, although she couldn't quite figure out why.

Meg Shaffer had known from the fourth month of her pregnancy that something would go wrong. That was when, at the age of twenty-four, she first went to work in an Intensive Care Nursery in Miami and suddenly became aware that not every pregnancy goes smoothly. "I was shocked to discover all the things that could happen," she told Stephanie.

"I never knew you worked in a nursery," Stephanie responded. "You told me you were a nurse, but you never mentioned the nursery."

"I guess I just didn't want to think about it much," Meg explained. "In school we learned the basic things about maternity nursing, but I was pretty surprised to find out how many babies are born prematurely, and how they almost always develop RDS—respiratory distress syndrome. It's really common. And learning that scared me a lot. I started taking better care of myself, like taking my vitamins and eating the right things and everything."

"Weren't you doing that before?"

"Not regularly. But when I went to work in the nursery I started worrying about all those things. I became aware of every little thing. I became aware of the fact the baby might not have moved for five hours, and I'd think, 'Oh my gosh! Something's wrong!' Or if it moved too much I'd think there was something wrong. And I was sure it was going to be a breach birth. And nurses in the nursery would say, 'Oh, you look like you're carrying real low for your first baby,' so of course I'd start thinking I was carrying too low. Most women with their first babies carry really high. So I went to my doctor and asked him why I was carrying the baby so low. He told me it might be breach, but then he said he was pretty sure it wasn't."

"You must have been going crazy," said Stephanie.

"She was," said Andy, taking his wife's hand.

"Every week I was sure there was something different wrong with me."

"You sound like a med student I used to know," said Stephanie, laughing as she recalled the young man who each week was convinced he had a different terminal illness.

"I was," Meg continued. "When we finally came up here I went for a sonogram. I was only thirty-three weeks pregnant but the head measurement came out at thirty-seven weeks, so I was convinced the baby was hydrocephalic—that he had an enlarged head caused by fluid buildup in the skull. For two weeks I couldn't sleep and I went to a specialist about it. He said there was nothing wrong and to go home and stop worrying myself to death. He told me last Friday that the baby seemed to be perfectly healthy, but that she would be big and could come at any time. But I've always had this feeling."

"What kind of specialist was he?" Stephanie asked.

"He was an obstetrician, but they say he's the best in Washington for sonograms. He went over every piece of the baby for me, its kidneys and the cord and heart—to see if it had four chambers—and everything was great. So then I was relieved."

"I'll bet!"

"Well, I thought, 'This baby's going to be fine, and everything's great,' but I still had the feeling the baby was going to come early, and I told everybody that. At Thanksgiving time I told my mother, 'I'm not carrying this baby more than two weeks longer.' I missed by two weeks. She was due January 15, but I had her December 24."

"Why did they have to do a section?" Stephanie wondered.

"God! That was just another thing to add to all my worries. Here I thought I was going to have a normal delivery because the doctor in Florida told me I would. Then the doctor here said, 'You're going to have to have a section because your pelvis is abnormal.' Then, when I was all worked up about that, another doctor said, 'No, your pelvis is fine. You'll have a normal delivery.' But when we got here they said, 'You're going to have to have a section.' So my head's been bouncing back and forth trying to prepare for this. Am I going to have a sore belly or a sore bottom? So I ended up with a section, which I wasn't too prepared for, and they really scared me, because being a nurse, I've seen a lot of surgical patients and I know the things that can go wrong."

"Were you totally out of it when the baby was born?"

"Oh, no. I saw the baby. For a second. And then they whisked her away, so I knew something was wrong."

"I heard two slurps," Andy told Stephanie, an indication that the baby had swallowed or aspirated some amniotic fluid during birth. Andy didn't know what the noise meant, but Meg had a pretty good idea what it was.

"I knew that it had probably aspirated while it was inside me, so I had a good premonition it probably had . . ."

"It was like two big gulps it took down," interrupted Andy, obviously proud of his powers of observation.

"I figured it probably would get aspiration pneumonia," continued Meg, a condition that can occur when fluid is taken into the lungs. "I knew they'd have to suction it out and I asked if there was any meconium, but they told me the fluid was clear. Then I figured I didn't have to worry about having a septic baby, so everything was all right that way. And Andy kept running around saying 'She's fine! She's fine! ' I was just sitting down here worrying about myself and the pain and everything and then the neonatologist came down and I got a creepy feeling as soon as he walked in."

As soon as Jim Hannan had begun to tell Meg and Andy that their baby had idiopathic respiratory syndrome, commonly referred to as respiratory distress syndrome, or RDS, Meg knew he wasn't just talking about a minor problem, and Hannan quickly realized he wasn't talking to just another middle-class mother. "He told me the baby was grunting," Meg told Stephanie, "and then I asked him if she was retracting, how fast was the respiration, and he said, 'Have you ever worked in a nursery? You seem familiar with this.' I said, 'Yes, I used to work in a nursery,' and then he just laid it right out on the line. Because I knew the baby could—could—" she hesitated, as though to say the word was to ensure its inevitability—"die. You could make it sound like nothing, but I knew and he knew I knew. It turns out it's not too serious," she continued, not sounding very convinced.

"When I went up to the nursery I asked the nurse how it was going and she said, 'Oh, you just have a little respiratory distress,' you know," said Andy. "And I thought that meant like a little shock, or just some minor thing, and I came down and told Meg and she just, well, it hit her hard because she knew what it was."

"I burst out crying," Meg confessed to Stephanie, with a little half-smile of embarrassment.

"Oh, God. Was this before the doctor had spoken to you?" asked Stephanie.

"Yes."

"She knew what RDS was and I didn't," Andy told his wife's friend.

"They don't like to call it hyaline membrane disease anymore," explained Meg.

"But that's what it is," Andy cut in. Hyaline membrane disease, which became familiar to the general public when it killed John F. Kennedy's third child, Patrick, is the disease described in the nursery as idiopathic respiratory syndrome. The diagnosis, however, cannot be finally made unless the baby dies and an autopsy is performed. Thus the term hyaline membrane disease is only used if the baby dies. But the symptoms—difficult breathing caused by immaturity of the premature baby's lungs, which collapse because they lack surfactant, the biochemical solution that gives mature lungs their elasticity—are the same no matter what the condition is called.

"So you assumed the worst?" Meg's friend asked.

"I did. She was on the respirator on thirty percent oxygen and it could have gone up, because they kept checking the oh-two levels, and, depending on the value, they'd increase the oxygen or decrease it. Andy was just up and he said they've decreased it all the way—she's on room air now. But sometimes these babies will go all the way to room air and then back on the respirator again. I've seen babies they've been playing that game with for five days before they finally get 'em well. Our baby was really lucky. I mean, the neonatologist came down and told me 'You have to expect the worst, even though it probably won't happen.'

"So I knew what was going to happen and of course I assumed the worst. And he," here she reached out for Andy's hand, "kept going up and coming back down and telling me 'There's nothing really wrong with it, it looks fine, it looks fine.' Well, I started believing him and relaxing a little, but then . . ."

"Is something else wrong?"

"No. But just when I was starting to relax a bit the neonatologist came back down and reminded me that the baby could have jaundice afterward. And they have to work on this problem and that problem and it probably won't go home with me. Then I figured there must be something else wrong because I'm going home Thursday, and that's seven days in the ICN, a long time for the baby to be there. But then I realized he was just reminding me of the worst that could happen, and it probably won't."

"He said that if he told us a date we'd hold him to it and take the baby away from them," Andy explained to Stephanie, who by that point was wishing she hadn't come and could find some graceful way to leave. She couldn't, so she plunged ahead.

"When are you going to go up and see her? And what's her name, for heaven's sake? You keep calling her it!"

"Alicia, Alicia Blackwood Shaffer," replied Meg. "I guess I'm sort of nervous about using her name and talking about her positively until I'm sure everything's all right. I know that sounds weird, but I saw too many mothers with babies in the nursery get attached to them and then lose them. I just can't help it."

"I don't think that sounds weird at all," Stephanie consoled her friend. "I mean, here you are expecting a bouncing, pink-cheeked baby, and then this. But you are going to go see her, aren't you?"

"Oh, sure. But I want to wait until the morning. Then I'll feel a lot better about everything. And I may not sound it, but this dope they've got me on is making me feel pretty strange. I want my head on straight before I have to go up there. We have a priest coming at the crack of dawn to baptize her, so I'll go up then."

"They're going to baptize her in the nursery? Isn't that a little early?"

"I suppose it is. But we arranged for it, or I should say Andy did, about three hours after she was born, when we weren't sure how things were going to go. Some nurse had told him she had a seventy-five percent chance of living. Andy told my mother that when he called her and she said, 'Get it baptized.' A little while later the hospital chaplain came down to see me and I said to myself, 'Mmm, things must not be going too well.' Anyway, I thought it would be nice to have her baptized right away. Especially since it's Christmas and everything. And the chaplain was so nice and gave us a lot of moral support, after that initial shock of seeing him walk in. It's nice because we don't have any family here, and you're the only good friend we've got in the area. The doctors have been really nice, but they're always in a hurry. The nurses too. They don't have time to just sit here and listen."

"I don't know how you did it," Stephanie said.

"Did what?

"Worked around those sick babies all the time. Wasn't it hard?"

"Yes. But I loved it. If we hadn't come here for Andy's new job I would have stayed there forever. I really liked that job. I hope I can find a job in an ICN up here, too."

"What was it you liked about it?"

"Well, I liked working with babies, and it was a real challenge for a nurse because you got to do a little bit more thinking . . ."

"With babies?"

"Yes. You got to make your own judgments. The babies are so dependent on you, and you really have to know them and try to anticipate their needs a lot more than you would for an adult patient. Any type of intensive care nursing is more of a challenge."

"But why the nursery? I'd think that if you were going to have children it would be an awful place to work. Wouldn't you rather work in an adult intensive care unit?" asked Stephanie, whose knowledge of hospitals was limited to two visits to an emergency room, one for a case of the flu and the other for a broken ankle.

"This may sound dumb," said Meg, "but part of it is, the patients are so big in an adult unit that the physical labor of trying to take care of them gets to be too hard. And sometimes you have a comatose patient, or whatever, and you have to turn them, and I can't do that because I have a bad back. I mean, I think the challenge could be just as great, and you do a lot of incredible nursing with adults, but I just can't do it physically. I worked on a surgical floor and we had a lot of sick people coming up from surgery. You had to use a lot of muscles and I'd end up with terrific backaches. So I decided to work with little people."

"But don't the sick babies get to you after a while? God! I know I could never work around babies like that. I'd flip out!" exclaimed Stephanie, who worked as an administrative assistant for a Northern Virginia congressman.

"I think it was starting to get to me," admitted Meg, who was beginning to look as though her Demerol was getting to her. "To be honest, I think I was beginning to get depressed."

"Wasn't that because you were pregnant?" Andy asked.

"I don't know if it was that. But right before I left the nursery we had a baby die. Remember?"

Andy nodded.

"Well, it was the first baby I'd seen die and that really made me sad."

"How long had the baby been there?" Stephanie asked.

"Just one night. It was a transport. We had gone to a community hospital to pick it up."

"What does something like that do to everybody?" asked Stephanie, who felt guilty for continuing the conversation in such a morbid vein but was unable to contain her curiosity.

"Well, first he was on a respirator, and we had to go through this big thing about whether we should turn it off. And it affected me a lot because I had never seen a dead baby before and when I saw what was happening, I thought I would faint. And the other nurses taking care of it were very upset, too. But the nurses who had been there a year or two years weren't fazed in the least—at least they didn't act like it. But I asked them to put up a screen so I wouldn't have to watch it. And when it died, this nurse put it in a garbage bag. I just couldn't believe it!" Meg's voice began to crack, and she was visibly upset as she thought about that pitiful bundle in the tan plastic bag. "You couldn't even tell it was a baby because of the garbage bag."

"Where did they put it after that?" asked Andy, who was hearing this part of the story for the first time. "They have to bury it, right?"

"No. They usually take it down to the morgue. And get this: We asked the parents what they wanted us to do with the body, where they wanted us to send it. They said, 'We don't want it. You keep it.' They were really poor and they didn't want to pay for a funeral. And they said, 'We'll give it to the university.' But the university didn't want it."

"What did you do with it?" Stephanie asked.

"Well, the doctor came in and asked the nurses if all of us wanted to take the baby's body into the back room and . . ." She paused for a moment, her smooth, pale, face flushing with embarrassment, ". . . this is really awful, but he wanted to know if we wanted to take the body into the back room and practice intubating it. Nurses aren't really trained to intubate babies, and we're usually not allowed to, so we never got to try on a live baby. But they wanted us to know how to do it in case we ever had to do it in an emergency. And since we worked with a lot of residents who knew much less than nurses did anyway, we really should have known how to do it."

"My God!" cut in Stephanie. "You didn't do it, did you?"

"No. I couldn't do it. Nobody could. But the next day, I told this one nurse who had been there for two years what had happened. I said, 'Do you know what Doctor Arnold wanted us to do? He wanted us to intubate that dead baby.' And she actually said, 'Why didn't you? I would have loved to do that myself.' I said, 'Well, if that's where you're at—but I couldn't do it.' Dead bodies give me the creeps, whether they're young or old. Just to go and . . . I just couldn't. Maybe later on, if I'm ever a nurse long enough. But after only three months with babies I couldn't do it."

"And you still want to work in a nursery?" Stephanie asked in amazement.

"Oh, yes."

"But why keep going if it bothered you that much?"

"Because I enjoyed it. At certain times it would get tense, and you'd feel sad, and you'd think about the babies . . ." She paused again. "I don't know if it's just me, or if a lot of nurses do it, but I was always thinking about those babies at home. I'm terrible to live with because I'm always at my job, even when I'm supposed to be home with Andy." Her husband nodded vigorously but smiled at the same time.

"She'd call the nursery and ask, 'How's baby so-and-so doing?' " Andy told Stephanie.

"I was always doing that. And on my day off I'd spend the time wondering whether a particular baby lived or died. If it was a really bad baby I'd have to know. I was always calling them up. So it does get to me. But I enjoy it too, because I think it's such an important job. And they need good, conscientious people to work with the babies because you can't make a mistake with newborns. You can make a medication error with an adult, and chances are, unless they're totally allergic to the medication, they're not going to die. But you make a little, itty, bitty mistake with a baby and that baby could die.

"We had one baby in the ICN—" she paused again for a moment, and then backtracked to better set the scene. "We had a lot of residents there. Here, upstairs, they have Fellows, which makes me feel a lot better. But we had mostly residents. And we even had some first-year residents who didn't have any idea what they were doing. Well, I had this one baby I was taking care of, a real little premie who had been on the respirator and then had been weaned off and was in an Isolette and was getting better. But they had ordered IVs and, instead of ordering .28 milligrams of magnesium for his body weight run into the IVs along with everything else, this resident ordered 2.8, which was a lot more than the baby needed. And as I was sitting there watching it, the baby's heart rate went down to about 80 or 90—usually it's around 160—and I couldn't understand why. The day before, I had taken care of the baby and its heart rate had been fine. Well, just then the mother came in to visit her baby and she said, 'My baby's so listless.' You know how mothers pick up on things a lot faster than most people? So I told the doctor and he grabbed the IV bottle on the stand and looked at it, and then he said, 'What's in this bottle?' He realized he had made a mistake and luckily picked up on it right away. If the kid had stayed on that fluid it could have just gone out. If the monitors hadn't been working— like sometimes when they go off you get really irritated and just turn the alarm off and forget to turn it back on—that baby could have gone down to zero and you wouldn't hear an alarm. If someone had turned that alarm off and that baby's heart rate had dropped, he probably would have died. And that's why it's really important to have good nurses, and I think I'm a good nurse."

"But that kind of thing doesn't happen much, does it?" asked Stephanie.

"Well, it doesn't happen that much, but when it does, you can have a dead baby. In the three months I was in the nursery we came across several problems with residents who didn't know what they were doing. One time, when I was taking care of this baby on a respirator, I had turned the baby over to change its position and the endoctracheal tube flipped from its trachea into its esophagus and its stomach started to blow up from the air being pumped in by the respirator. I knew the tube was out of place, but technically, inserting tubes and taking them out is a resident's job. I wasn't supposed to do it. So I called the resident and when she came in I told her the tube wasn't in place. Well, she looked at the baby with his stomach swelling up and said, 'Oh, I think it's in place. The baby's just fighting the respirator.'

"I kept insisting that it wasn't in place," Meg continued, "and all the other nurses started coming around. This resident was new, but I was new too, so I was afraid to say, 'You stupid idiot! Take that out!' But I kept telling her 'It's not in right.' Now I know I should have yanked it myself, and I feel bad that I didn't. Well, the baby's stomach started swelling up like this," she said, placing her hands under the sheet and raising it up like a balloon over her abdomen. "The baby turned blue and the heart rate went down to about 60, so they were doing CPR [cardio-pulmonary resuscitation] on it and everything. I picked up the phone and called a Fellow, but this resident wasn't doing anything! Not a thing. She was just standing there!"

"You're kidding!" said Stephanie, who was having a hard time believing what she was hearing.

"No. She just didn't know what to do. If you're in doubt, pull the tube. That's the rule. If in doubt, pull the tube. And she wouldn't because she was scared she couldn't put one back in. She had never put a tube in before, so she was scared that if she pulled it out she wouldn't be able to reinsert it, and the baby had to be on a respirator. So meanwhile, this kid blew up into a balloon and almost burst. Finally the Fellow, who had been in another part of the hospital, came running in, took one look, and yanked the tube. She reinserted it in the trachea and the baby was fine."

"What happened to the resident?" asked Andy.

"The Fellow gave her a good yelling and talking to, and then she came over to us nurses and said, 'I know you're not technically supposed to pull tubes or anything, but pull the tube! When in doubt, pull the tube. The residents we get around here sometimes are not the hottest, and you're just going to have to take over.' Well, this got the nurses pissed off and we said we didn't think they should have incompetent people in charge of the nursery, risking the lives of the babies. It was after that that they wanted us to practice inserting the endotracheal tube in the dead baby. You just can't insert tubes and lines on the spur of the moment if you haven't been taught how to do it properly. And they sure didn't teach us how to work with two-pound babies in nursing school."

"Talk about taking your work home. We left there three months ago and she still worries about those babies," said Andy. "Meg practically brought her work to Washington with her."

"That must be rough on a marriage," said Stephanie.

"It's really hard to be a husband of anyone in the medical profession," Andy replied, "a doctor or a nurse. But now that I've 'nursed' her for just eight hours I can understand what she does, and I can't complain now, because she's really doing a good thing working like that all the time.

"But when did you see each other?"

"We never did."

"Weekends were the best," said Andy, "because during the

week she'd only work three days and then I'd see her two. And then on weekends we'd have the daytime. I guess the whole thing was really pretty terrible."

"He's a real good husband," said Meg, smiling at Andy, " 'cause he's flexible. A lot of people might not put up with it. But he has to understand that it's my profession and I have a right to do what I like. I do want to progress in this, not just work a couple of days a week for the rest of my life. I want to go back full time, try to get my masters and stay in neonatology."

"But don't nurses get pushed into administration if they get a masters?" Stephanie asked.

"Not necessarily. You could get pushed into teaching, which would be fun. I don't really want to do staff nursing all my life. Nobody can handle that for very long. It's exhausting, and working nights and evenings is just not practical if you have a family. Right now I can swing it, and I'll manage it with one baby. But if I had any more I wouldn't be able to do it."

"You could always do it part time," said Andy. "That's one of the practical things about nursing. You can always work a few days a week."

"But one of the bad things," countered Meg, "is that patients just don't stop needing you at three o'clock, or whenever the shift's over. He has a nine-to-five job," she said of her statistician husband, "and at five he just gets up and leaves. Well, for the first six months of our marriage he just didn't understand that I couldn't always leave when the shift was supposed to be over. If a patient needs you, or there's other work that just has to be done, you stay. It's that simple. It was hard for him to understand that for a while. But now he realizes that if someone needs to go to the bathroom at eleven, you don't just say, 'Sorry, I'm off duty now; I can't help you.' And the same thing applies to babies. Sometimes they might all of the sudden spit up all over the place just as you're about to get off. Well, you can't just leave the baby lying there where he could aspirate."

"What made me mad was that I'd go to pick her up and I'd have to wait two hours in the parking lot," said Andy.

"Speaking of waiting," said Stephanie, "what time is it? I was supposed to meet someone at Clyde's at eleven to toast in Christmas. I've really got to get out of here."

"Thanks a lot for coming over, Steph. We were feeling so alone here. And it's really cheered me up to be able to talk about some of this stuff. I mean it."

"I didn't come here to drag all this out of you," Stephanie began as she pulled on her coat.

"You didn't," replied Meg. "I think I've kept a lot of this to myself for too long. I'm really grateful to you for listening."

"Any time. As a matter of fact, I'd like to come back tomorrow to see the baby. What time's the baptism? Maybe I could come for that."

"Seven A.M.," replied Andy, rising from his chair by the head of Meg's bed.

"In that case I think I'll pass," said Stephanie, laughing. "But I will come by later in the day. Merry Christmas, you two. I know everything will work out fine."

"Merry Christmas, Stephie. And thanks again," said Meg, whose eyelids were beginning to flutter.

"Wait up, Stephanie. I'll walk you to the elevator," called Andy as Stephanie walked out the door.

"I'll be right back, honey. I want to go see Alicia again and then I'll come back and say good night." He leaned over and kissed his wife gently on the forehead.

"Hurry back," she said, "or I'll be asleep before you get here."

Chapter Twelve

The arrival of the night shift at 11 P.M. caused the day's most radical and obvious transformation in mood and atmosphere in the nursery. The nurses seemed to sweep into the ICN, laughing and talking loudly among themselves. There was shouting from one section of the nursery to another, shouting to carry on long-distance conversations, rather than call someone to the phone, or call for help. The coffee urn, which had remained in the nurses' lounge for sixteen hours, suddenly appeared on a counter in Room 445. During the day there was not so much as a cup of coffee in the ICN, although the cups would begin appearing during the evening shift. And, as Jessica Durand had suspected, one of the young women made a beeline for the tape recorder sitting on top of Stephen's Isolette and, taking a tape from a small box she had brought to work with her, instantly filled the three rooms with the sounds of the Eagles. The music was all the more startling because, for the first time that day or evening, the heart-beat rhythms of the monitors and the shrill scolding of the alarms were no longer the predominant sounds in the three rooms.

Donna Zeeman, the head nurse on the shift, had no sooner taken off her coat, scrubbed, and made a quick visual survey of the three rooms than she was on the phone to the hospital's night director of nursing. "Harriett? Donna. Thanks, Merry Christmas to you, too. Listen, Harriett, it sure as hell isn't going to very merry up here if we can't get at least one more body. I go home for eighteen hours and come back to find we've got two new babies on respirators and one of them looks sick as hell. Sure I know what night this is! You think this is where I want to be? But these babies don't give a damn why we're short-handed. I've only got seven girls tonight and I have to have eight. No. Everybody's either out of town or tied up. I know what their plans are because I checked Wednesday to see if there was anyone I could call in case something like this happened. No. There's no one. Haven't you got somebody down on OB you could give us? Well, we could put her in step down and move Ingrid into A or B. You haven't got anybody? Terrific! No, I know. I'll just have to see what we can do." She slammed the receiver down. "Shit!" Donna exploded. "I don't care what the hell her problems are, we can't take care of these babies properly with only seven people!"

"Call Mabel," suggested Darlene Michaelson, one of the old hands on the shift. "She'll come up with someone."

"I hate to call her now. It's almost midnight and it's Christmas Eve. But . . ."

"Call her!" urged Robin English, a nurse who was still young enough to derive a certain warped pleasure from the idea of having the boss called at home late at night.

"All right. I guess we don't have much choice," said Donna. "Darlene, check the number for me, will you?" she asked the woman, who was sitting at the desk in the entrance area.

Darlene flipped through the listing of home phone numbers

until she came to that for Mabel Parrington, the nurse coordinator for the ICN.

"Hello. Jack Parrington? Donna Zeeman. I'm terribly sorry to disturb you and hope I didn't wake you . . . I didn't? Thank God! But is Mabel there? Thanks. . . . They were awake," she whispered to Darlene.

"Damn!" muttered the young nurse, and two of the other nurses, who were standing beside her, began to giggle. Donna made a *shhhhhhsh*ing motion with her hand.

"Mabel. Listen, I'm really sorry to be calling like this. Yes, we do. We've only got seven girls and we've got two new respirator babies. Right. And one of them's really sick. I tried that. I haven't got anybody I can call in tonight, and I called Harriett. Not a soul. Right. I'm really sorry, but I felt we had to. Okay. I hope we don't." She hung up the phone and then bellowed, "Now hear this! I want this coffee urn out of here and back where it belongs and I want that music turned down! Shape up, ladies, Mabel's coming in!"

"You're kidding," said Robin English.

"I would not kid about something like this," said Donna.

"Cripes! Why tonight?" complained Annie Miller. "It's bad enough being here on Christmas without having the brass here, too."

The night crew was really something of an unknown quantity for Mabel Parrington. She had spent one night on about three months earlier, because there had been some complaints from parents about the noise level and irreverence. But there hadn't been anything Mabel could put her finger on when she was there. Obviously, she'd thought, the nurses had all been on their best behavior. But she was sure the women of the night shift knew their nursing. The tests had proven that. All the nurses in the unit had gone through a series of what were called in-service tests, and the night shift had done extremely well. So at least lack of skill wasn't a problem. It was just that there was no question the 11-to-7 shift attracted some "different" people.

Mabel had never had any problem understanding why someone would work evenings, particularly married nurses with young children. That was logical. A difficult way of life, perhaps, but logical. Midnights, however, were a different matter. That was a little weird. But as long as they knew their nursing, gave the babies good care, and came through in the clutch—all of which they did continually—she wasn't about to rock the boat by probing too deeply into individual reasons for wanting to be on the shift.

One nurse who didn't seem part of the night-shift group but at the same time could fit without being noticed into any of the shifts was Ingrid Obst, an older woman who worked in the C section with the babies who were generally just a step away from discharge or return to the regular nursery. Ingrid was a quiet woman who, with her husband, had come to the United States as a refugee after World War II. She, perhaps more than anyone else in the nursery, was constantly grappling internally with the social and ethical questions raised by society's paying as much as $100,000 to provide life-saving care for babies who, it sometimes seemed, were only being saved for a life of poverty, despair, and, she feared, crime.

There were others in the nursery who, at least in their darker moments, shared Ingrid's opinions. But when they thought about the situation long enough they would realize that, even if society provided no care for these babies, some of them would live. And those who did live would be far sicker, and cost society far more in the long run, if they were given no care at birth. Additionally, Jim Hannan always liked to remind anyone who would listen that the sickest babies represented only the tip of the iceberg. A commitment by society to care for those who seemingly had the poorest chance of survival inevitably filtered down into better care for those who started off with a better chance. And conversely, a social attitude that denied help to the weakest often denied help to those not so weak, who could derive even more benefit from the help.

Ingrid was more of a fixture at Metropolitan Lying-In than the Intensive Care Nursery in which she worked. Having begun her career at the hospital twenty-seven years ago, she remembered the days when there was no real ICN, and the area in which she now worked was occupied by operating rooms, not Isolettes. She had spent most of her years working in the labor and delivery rooms and on the adult floors, caring for both OB and gynecology patients. But about five years ago she had decided to "slow down," as she told friends—moving to the nursery where she felt the patients were easier to care for. Despite the pressures and tension of the ICN, Ingrid's view was shared by many of the nurses, particularly the younger ones. For many nurses feel that infants, no matter how sick, are easier patients than adults: They can be turned and moved without any physical strain; they can be forced to take medication without argument; they don't talk back; they don't question the nurse's authority to make them do whatever the nurse tells them to do. At the same time, however, Ingrid was quite different from her younger colleagues in that she wanted less, rather than more, authority and responsibility. While many of the ICN nurses liked the work because of the atmosphere of cooperation and responsibility shared with the physicians, Ingrid liked it because there were always physicians in the ICN, or moments away, and she could turn all the decisions and problems over to them. But then, she'd say, "If you put twenty-seven years in a hospital behind you, you have a little wear and tear behind you and want to slow down."

As she was approaching her own retirement, the older nurse began to question all the money being spent to save the lives of tiny prematures, while she could see the elderly getting short shrift from society. She would sit in one of the nursery rockers, feeding a baby, and silently watch as the parents, many of them on welfare and some of them young children themselves, would come to visit their babies. "I wonder why we should pay for this," the old woman would often think, disgusted. "We have old people we have to take care of. My time to quit has almost come. I've been paying my taxes and my money goes to support these people. All my life I've been in services to help people, and what's left for me? When my husband or I go out and we need a pair of glasses, we pay for the glasses. If *we* had Medicaid, that would pay for them." Her thoughts would drift back to the immediate postwar days in Germany, when society was in chaos and "everybody comes back from the war—soldiers, nurses, everybody—and there's two thousand people for every job. But *I* found a job, because *I* looked for a job. I didn't get what I wanted, but I got a job. I did what I could. I worked as a cashier in a restaurant where the GIs came in. These people could get a job," she would think. "There are jobs. It's just whether you want it."

Ingrid thought about the young mother she had spoken with a few weeks earlier. She had exchanged pleasantries with the girl a few times and finally had to ask, "How old are you?"

"I'm sixteen," the girl replied.

"And who is taking care of your baby when he goes home?" Ingrid asked, her German accent and syntax probably as hard for Washington blacks to cut through as was their dialect for her.

"I will," the girl told her.

"But you say you are only sixteen. Won't you go back to school?"

"I'm gonna go nights for a while."

"What about your mother? You live with her?"

The girl nodded.

"Is your mother not going to help you?" asked Ingrid.

"My mother's in college. She ain't got no time."

And there the conversation ended. "My God," Ingrid thought. "Here is a woman who is trying to get ahead. She probably started like her daughter and now she is making something of herself. And then her daughter does something like this." She slowly shook her head in wonder and anger dulled by years of hearing similar stories. There was no question, she felt, that these parents seemed to care about their tiny babies. But there was such a lack of reality to that care. Parents would want to take the babies out of the Isolettes or cribs for long periods of time and would not seem to understand why they had to put them back. Ingrid would say, "You can't keep the baby out for so long. The baby gets cold, the baby gets sick." But the child-parents would simply stare at her, uncomprehending. And then what, she would wonder, would become of these babies the babies would be taking home with them?

"Ingrid?"

"Yes. Oh, good evening, Dr. Noble," replied the nurse, who had not, despite herself, been able to shake the years of formality in nurse-physician relationships she had picked up in other areas of the hospital.

"Hi. Listen, Ingrid, I'm about to go up to the residents' room and try to get a few hours' sleep. Don't call me for every little thing, okay? Wait until you have a few IVs that need restarting and then wake me up." He winked at Ingrid, who smiled in return. "Good night, ladies! Merry Christmas to all, and to all a good night!" Noble called, blowing a kiss into the nursery as he walked out—and just missed bumping into Mabel Parrington, who had walked in and was pulling off her coat.

"Excuse me, Mabel! Good night, Mabel. I'll be upstairs if you need me and I hope you don't," said Noble, scurrying off toward the stairs.

"Good night, John," replied Mabel, too startled to say much else.

The rock music level was tolerable when Mabel Parrington arrived in the nursery at 1 A.M. Unpleasant, she thought, but she had worked this shift on a few occasions before, just to see what was going on, and had decided that there was no way to avoid the music, given the number of youngsters on the shift. It wasn't that there weren't enough senior people with experience, but the night shift seemed to draw a large proportion of women under twenty-five. The only good thing about the night shift in the ICN, Mabel often thought, was that she had managed to make it largely voluntary. There were enough experienced nurses who wanted the strange hours, as well as enough beginners, so that she rarely had to draft staff for the overnight stint.

"Hi, Donna. Sorry I took so long getting in, but the car wouldn't start," Mabel told the shift supervisor.

"Hey, listen. I'm just sorry we had to bother you at home, tonight of all nights. Is it still snowing out?" Donna asked her boss.

"No. Some of the back roads are still pretty slippery, but the main ones aren't too bad. Okay. Who do you want me to take?"

"I guess baby Alvarez. But listen, we need to talk about this staffing problem."

"Not tonight, Donna. We'll get it worked out next week," Mabel told her. "Tonight let's just worry about making it to tomorrow morning."

As she went about suctioning the secretions from baby Alvarez's lungs and checking his monitor settings, Mabel observed the other staffers at work. What always amazed her when she'd come in like this was that the faces changed so rarely. The situation was the same on the day shift. But she was always too busy then to stop and think about it. Now, with the ICN devoid of parents, physicians, or any other distractions—besides the Eagles—she could think about her lack of a turnover problem. Most ICN nurse coordinators she had talked to, in Washington and in other areas of the country, reported that their nurses stayed an average of 1.8, at most two, years. But here at Metropolitan, most nurses stayed well beyond that. Some even remained in the ICN five years or more. She supposed much of it had to be attributed to Jim Hannan's attitude toward nurses. While on the one hand he terrorized them, on the other he gave them as much responsibility and opportunity to learn and grow as they wanted. He was well aware that the nurses were the backbone of the ICN. He was never upset to be called at home by a nurse second-guessing a physician, because nine times out of ten, the nurse was right and the doctor was wrong. In most settings, Mabel knew, particularly most non-intensive care settings, if a nurse called the director at home to complain about the medical judgments of a physician—well, she better have skills in another line of work.

Because the night was so filled with the critical minutiae of carring for a full load of babies, time passed quickly, with little of the usual nighttime chatter and visiting. John Noble was called downstairs at least once an hour, usually to restart IVs that had slipped out of the babies' doll-like hands. But when he came downstairs at 4:50 A.M., Noble took one look at baby boy Alvarez and decided it was time to give the boss a call. As was usually the case, the phone by Jim and Christie's bed was answered by the second ring.

"Ya?"

"Jim? John. I'm sorry to do this to you. But I think the time has come to decide what to do with Alvarez."

"What's up?"

"Nothing. Everything's down. His blood gases look much worse; he's even duskier, if that's possible, and sweaty. I think we may be moving toward congestive heart failure and, if the kid arrests, I'd feel better if we already had our decisions made."

"You're right," Hannan told him. "Frankly, I was going to get up at 5:30 anyway. If I didn't, the kids would tear all the packages apart before I even got down. You've just sped things along a bit. I'll see you in twenty minutes."

"You can't get down here that fast; there's snow on the road."

"Right. Make it twenty-five minutes."

Chapter Thirteen

Thirty minutes later Jim Hannan was standing beside the warming table on which baby boy Alvarez lay. Hannan didn't think the baby looked much worse than he had about ten hours earlier. But what was more important, he did not look any better. His skin was still an unreal shade of blue-gray. His enormous chest rose and fell rhythmically, precisely in time to the Bourns Infant Respirator that stood beside the warming table. Hannan was going over the chart when John Noble walked up to him.

"Merry Christmas, Jim."

"It's not gonna be very merry for this little sucker or his parents, I'm afraid. I disagree with your thought that he looks worse, but these numbers—" he gestured toward the last lab report in the chart—"say you're right and I'm wrong. I guess the time has come. . . . Has the mother been up at all yet to see him?"

"No."

202

"Well, I'd better go downstairs and get this over with," he thought. "No point in dragging it out." He banged the chart and its clipboard down sharply on the warming table with a loud *crack!* Noble and the two nurses in the room turned to look at him, startled. But baby boy Alvarez, his tiny brain fogged by morphine, didn't move. "Shit!" exclaimed Hannan, quietly and bitterly at the same time. Was this what he went to medical school for? Was this why he trained longer than a neurosurgeon? So that he could tell a woman there wasn't a thing he could do to save her firstborn child? He strode quickly from the nursery, stripping off his gown and tossing it in the basket near the door as he left the room.

Hannan didn't hear the half-dozen "Merry Christmas, Doctor's" he received on his way down to Room 345, and he didn't see the artificial Christmas trees and hokey decorations at each of the nursing stations. All he could think about was how much he hated this part of the job he loved, and how it was no easier this time than it had been about a dozen times before.

The irony was that, while Hannan was dreading telling Maria and Raoul Alvarez that it was time to let their son complete the dying process begun with his birth twenty hours earlier, they were panicked by the thought that he might tell them something else. Maria had lain awake most of the night and slept fitfully when she had slept at all, remembering bits and pieces of the newspaper acounts of the Karen Ann Quinlan case. What if Hannan, like the doctors treating the twenty-one-year-old comatose New Jersey woman, refused to give up? What if he said he could not turn off the respirator, for fear of the law? Would her baby lie on that table Raoul had told her about, just lie there for weeks, for months, suffering? Would she and Raoul, like the Quinlans, have to hire a lawyer and go to court to plea for their baby's death? Would . . .

"Mrs. Alvarez?" Hannan rapped on the door frame and stuck his head into the room. "May I come in?" he asked, shyly she thought.

"Yes, Doctor Hannan, of course. Come in," Maria Alvarez replied. Hannan was pleased to see she was sitting up in bed, the pillows propping her up. Her short black hair was neatly brushed and she had put on a bit of makeup. She was clearly pulled together, and not at all in the kind of semihysterical shape the physician was afraid he might find her in.

"I've just been to see the baby," Hannan told the parents, "and I'm afraid the news isn't good."

"There's been no improvement?" Raoul Alvarez asked.

"No. The baby's essentially the same as he was when we spoke last night. If anything he's gotten a bit worse. His breathing is slightly more difficult than it was before. Do you have any questions about him?"

"No," said Maria, speaking for herself and her husband, who sat beside the bed, holding his wife's hand and looking up at the doctor who stood at the foot of the bed. "I think it is time for you to stop," Maria told Hannan, giving voice to the words she had repeated to herself throughout the night.

"I agree with you," Hannan told her, and for the first time he saw tears in her eyes. But they were tears of relief as much as they were tears of sorrow.

"Don't worry, Doctor," said Maria Alvarez, dabbing at her cheeks with a tissue. "Our tragedy is not for our baby to die. Our tragedy is for our baby to be sick. My baby isn't living. The only time he was living was when he was inside of me. The rest of the time he is just artificially living, and that is not alive."

"There's not much more I can say," Hannan told her, "except, I just want to tell you again: If this were my baby I'd want what you want. I'll be down later to talk to you." He softly tapped the foot of the bed with his right hand as he stepped from the room before she could say thank you. He did not want to be thanked for what would come next.

"Have spent considerable time evaluating baby and speaking with parents," Hannan wrote in the chart when he reached the nursery. "They are very aware of the problems and the nil outlook for survival. We have decided to provide only supportive care and not including respirator or respiratory supplement. Parents have requested discontinuance of heroic support." He signed the note, "Hannan." This time he laid the chart down on the table gently, almost reverently. He then reached over with his left hand and flipped the switch, deactivating the alarm on the respirator. The beginning had ended and the end was beginning. The nursing notes tell the rest:

"6:10—Ventilator turned off by Dr. Hannan. Monitor discontinued by Dr. Hannan. Heart rate below 100 immediately and color became quite dusky."

Marian Barnes couldn't help thinking of her own three children as she wrote the note. A thirteen-year veteran of the nursery, she had pulled the death watch, a duty she was more than used to but always resented. "It's the right thing to do," she had to tell herself, as she sat behind the screen set up around the warming table. "It's best for the baby's sake and best for the parents' sake. He could never have hoped to lead a normal life . . ." She busied herself with nursery paperwork and tried not to think about the baby a few feet from her.

"6:25—Baby gasped three times between 6:10 and 6:25 and heart rate slow and faint.

"7—No heart rate. No respirations. Baby baptized by M. Barnes, RN.

"7—Baby pronounced dead by Dr. Noble. Measurements and footprints taken. Mother did not wish to see the baby. Baby taken to morgue. M. Barnes, RN."

Baby boy Alvarez, baptized Raoul in his last minutes of half-life, had lived seventeen hours and thirty-one minutes. His mother had never seen him. As she had said when her husband asked whether she wanted to visit the nursery, "Why see the baby if I cannot hold him?"

Once again Hannan returned to Room 345, leaving to Marian Barnes the job of bathing the baby, swaddling it in a blue disposable cloth, and placing it in a light tan plastic garbage bag for the trip to the basement morgue. He walked down the stairs slowly, thinking of an easy way to say, "Your baby is dead." But all he could think to say when he entered the room was just that: "Mrs. Alvarez, your baby is dead."

"Thank you, doctor. That is good news for us and our son," Maria Alvarez responded. This time she did not cry, and there was a slight, wistful smile on her lips. Hannan stood quietly, looking down at her, for at least two minutes. Then he turned quickly and left the room, hurrying back up to his office.

Noble was waiting for Hannan when the nursery director returned to the office. Hannan flung himself violently into his chair. "I can do without that shit!" He spat the words out, staring at his young colleague sitting on the couch.

"Don't be so hard on yourself, Jim," Noble said quietly, reversing their usual roles. "All you did was accept the inevitable. You just let nature take it's course."

"Bullshit! I killed that baby. I could have kept it going. I told one of the residents I could get an eggplant breathing if I could intubate it. But what would the point be? The kid wouldn't have ever left the table. I wanted that baby to die."

"You know," Hannan said very quietly, "I have a recurring dream every so often: I'm going to heaven, and as I go in through the gates I see what looks like this field of gently waving grass. When I look closely, it's babies, slowly undulating back and forth. The babies I've shut off."

Chapter Fourteen

Meg Shaffer wondered why the shades were drawn in the main nursery, but she didn't say anything to Andy as he pushed her wheelchair from the elevator to the door of Room 445. He had been warned to keep Meg out of the center room and had washed before going down to get her. He paused just inside the door to pull on one of the two gowns he had placed there a few minutes earlier. He helped Meg into hers and then wheeled her directly to Alicia's Isolette on the far wall.

Meg stared straight ahead, not wanting to see any of the other babies, attempting to block the cacophony of nursery sounds that immediately brought back the painful, rather than the good, memories of her ICN experience. She had thought the baptism, at least rushing it this way, was really a little silly. But as she heard the ticking of the monitors and the shrill scream of alarms, she decided she was doing the right thing.

As Andy pushed the wheelchair into place alongside Alicia's

Isolette, a woman he didn't recognize as one of the nurses or doctors stepped back out of the way.

"Mr. and Mrs. Shaffer?" inquired the woman, extending her right hand. "I'm Ellen Richardson, from St. Michael's."

"Yes?" responded Andy, who wasn't quite sure what was happening. When he had called yesterday afternoon the woman to whom he had spoken had promised the priest would be in the nursery by 7:15, the only time he could squeeze a hospital baptism into his schedule on Christmas Day. Here it was, 7:20, and Andy didn't see any priest, and the church hadn't said anything about anyone else coming over. "Is Father Richards here yet?" Andy asked the woman.

"It's Richardson," she said, smiling, "and I'm the 'Father.'"

"You're an Episcopal priest?"

"Yes, I'm the assistant rector of St. Michael's. Father Potter is busy preparing for the Christmas services, so I agreed to come over this morning. Do you or your wife have any problems with that?"

"Oh, no," Meg responded, looking up quickly from her daughter, whom she was seeing for the first time. Sensing Andy's confusion, Meg explained, "Where we come from everybody's still arguing about whether women should be ordained, and we've certainly never met a female priest before. But thank you for coming. This really means a lot to me—to us." She looked up at Andy and took his hand.

"Let's get started then, shall we," said Reverend Richardson, placing her white embroidered stole around her neck.

Alicia was sleeping on her back, her arms spread wide, a red monitor lead attached to her left thigh and a black lead protruding from her right chest. At just over 6¾ pounds she looked like a newborn Gulliver among neonatal Lilliputians.

"What we're going to do," said Reverend Richardson, picking up her prayerbook from the top of the Isolette, "is just have some prayers and some scriptures, and then the baptism itself." She was interrupted by the scream of Alicia's monitor, which

Andy silenced by pushing the reset button. "It keeps going off," he explained.

"Let's get started," said the priest. "There is one body and one Spirit, there is one hope . . ." The monitor went off with its ear-splitting *Eeeeeeee!* ". . .from God's call to us, one Lord, one faith, one baptism, one God and father of all.

"The Lord be with you. Let us pray. Heavenly Father, giver of life and health, comfort and renew thy servant, Alicia, and give your power of healing to those who minister to her needs, that she may be strengthened in her weakness and have confidence in your love and care. Through Jesus Christ, our Lord, who lives and reigns with you and the Holy Spirit, one God, now and forever, Amen." *Eeeeeeee!* Without lifting his eyes from the floor, Andy reached over and punched the reset button to silence the monitor.

As the service continued, Meg stared at her new daughter. "She isn't that bad," she thought, noting how peacefully Alicia was sleeping. "Her color's good; she's breathing well." Her eyes darted from the body to the monitor read-outs and back to her baby, continually checking the numbers that told her what was going on inside the sleeping infant. "I just can't believe I got so upset," she thought. "Now I feel kind of ridiculous going through with this. She's going to live." But then her thoughts drifted back to the nursery in which she had worked in Florida, and the large babies who had seemed to be doing so well and suddenly turned sour and died. And she began to listen to the words of the service.

"Let me read just one passage of scripture to you," said the priest. "This is from the Gospel of Mark, where Jesus blesses the little children. 'Some people brought children to Jesus for Him to place His hands on them, but the disciples scolded the people. And when Jesus noticed this He was angry and said to His disciples, Let the children come to Me and do not stop him . . .'" *Eeeeeeeeee!* "'. . . because the Kingdom of God belongs to such as these and I assure you that whosoever does not receive the

Kingdom of God like a child will never enter it. And then He took the children in His arms, placed His hands on each of them and blessed them.' " *Eeeeeeee!*

The business of the nursery continued around the trio gathered at the Isolette, as though baptisms were a daily event in the ICN. The day shift was replacing the night shift, "Merry Christmas's" were being exchanged liberally, and but for the general depression brought about by the death of Raoul Alvarez, nursery life was going on as it would any morning. The only sound Ellen Richardson seemed to notice, other than that of the alarms, was the ticking of the various cardiac monitors, for she sped up the service as though performing to a metronome of heart beats.

"He's saying that each of us is welcome in His arms," the priest continued. "Your daughter, Alicia Blackwood, always has a home there. The Lord invites her to come just as close as she wants to and invites her to climb into His arms, and you can trust that those arms are carrying her, holding her up, and strengthening her. I want you two to name your daughter. What is the name you have given her?"

"Alicia Blackwood," said Meg, wiping a tear from the corner of her left eye with one hand and stroking Alicia's foot inside the Isolette with the other.

"Will you be responsible for seeing that she is brought up in a Christian life?" the priest asked.

"I will with God's help," responded Meg, calling on her memories of years of Sunday services and baptisms. Her husband muttered the same reply.

"And will you by your prayers and witness help her to grow into the full stature of Christ?"

"I will with God's help," came the two voices in unison.

"Let's offer some prayers for her. Deliver her, O Lord, from the way of sin and death, open her heart to your grace and truth. Fill her with your holy and life-giving spirit. Keep her in faith and communion with your holy church, teach her to love others in the same spirit, send her into the world in witness to your love and bring her to the fullness of your peace. And grant, O Lord, that all who are baptized into the death of Jesus Christ your Son may live in the power of His resurrection, and look for Him to come again in Glory who lives and reigns . . ." *eeeeeeee!* ". . . now and forever. Amen.

"The Lord be with you."

"And also with you," responded Meg and Andy.

"Let us give thanks to the Lord our God."

"It is right to give Him praise and thanks," they both replied, watching their daughter sleep.

"We thank you, almighty God, for the gift of water," continued Reverened Richardson. "Over it the . . ." *eeeeeeee!* ". . . Holy Spirit moved in the beginning of creation. Through it you lead the children of Israel out of their bondage in Egypt into the land of promise. In it your Son, Jesus, received the baptism of John and was annointed by the Holy Spirit as the Messiah, the Christ, to lead us, through his death and resurrection, from the bondage of sin to everlasting life.

"We thank you, Father, for the water of baptism. In it we are buried with Christ in His death. By it we share in His resurrection. Through it we are reborn, by the Holy Spirit. Therefore, in joyful obedience to your Son, we bring into this fellowship those who come to Him in faith, baptizing them in the name of the Father, and of the Son, and of the Holy Spirit." With this Reverend Richardson reached forward and picked up a small dish filled with the holy water she had brought with her to the nursery. Then she said, "Now sanctify this water, we pray you, by the power of your Holy Spirit, that those who hear are cleansed from sin and born again and may continue forever in the risen life of Jesus Christ, our Saviour.

"To Him, to . . ." *eeeeeeee!* ". . . you, and to the Holy Spirit, be all honor and glory, now and forever. Amen. Alicia Blackwood," said the priest, dipping the first two fingers of her right hand in the holy water and reaching through a portal into the Isolette, "I baptize you in the name of the Father, and of the

Son, and of the Holy Spirit. Amen." Alicia stirred, squinted, and then slipped back into sleep as the drops of water touched her forehead in the sign of the cross. Meg could only look at the Kleenex she was busily working in her lap. Andy, who was standing behind Meg's wheelchair with his hands on her shoulders, just watched Alicia.

"Heavenly Father, we thank you that by water and the Holy Spirit you have bestowed on this your servant the forgiveness of sin and raised her to the new life of Grace. Sustain her, O Lord, in your Holy Spirit, to hold her in the arms of your mercy, to keep her safe with prayer.

"Give her an . . ." *eeeeeeee!* Reverend Richardson finally had to fight to hold back a giggle, as did Andy, ". . . inquiring and discerning heart, the courage to will and to persevere, a spirit to know and to love you, and the gift of joy and wonder in all your works. Amen."

Then reaching once again into the Isolette, Ellen Richardson gently traced a cross on Alicia's forehead with an oil-covered fingertip, saying, "Alicia, you are sealed by the Holy Spirit and marked as Christ's own forever. Amen."

"Now you're a child of God, you little rascal," said Andy Shaffer, reaching into the Isolette to stroke his daughter's cheek and then his wife's hand, which was resting on Alicia's legs. And in reaching in he set off the monitor once again, filling the corner of the nursery with a resounding *EEEEEEEEEEEEEEEEE-EEEEEE!*